D1078526

DR JOAN GOMEZ is Honorary Consulting Psychiatrist
to the Chelsea and Westminster Hospital. She was
trained at King's College, London, ~

MRCPsy   respectively. She was
elected Fellow of the Royal College of Psychiatrists in
1982, obtained the Diploma in the History of Medicine
in 1996, and the Diploma in the Philosophy of Medicine
in 1998. She is a Fellow of the Society of Apothecaries
and also of the Royal Society of Medicine. She has been
engaged in clinical work and research on the interface
between psychiatry and physical medicine. Dr Gomez is
also the author of five other books published by Sheldon
Press: *Coping with Thyroid Problems* (1994), *How to
Cope with Bulimia* (1995), *Living with Diabetes* (1995),
How to Cope with Anaemia (1998), and *Living with
Crohn's Disease* (2000). Her husband was a general
practitioner and they have ten children.

Overcoming Common Problems Series

For a full list of titles please contact
Sheldon Press, Marylebone Road, London NW1 4DU

The Assertiveness Workbook
A plan for busy women
JOANNA GUTMANN

Birth Over Thirty Five
SHEILA KITZINGER

Body Language
How to read others' thoughts by their gestures
ALLAN PEASE

Body Language in Relationships
DAVID COHEN

The Cancer Guide for Men
HELEN BEARE AND NEIL PRIDDY

Cider Vinegar
MARGARET HILLS

Comfort for Depression
JANET HORWOOD

Coping Successfully with Panic Attacks
SHIRLEY TRICKETT

Coping Successfully with Your Irritable Bowel
ROSEMARY NICOL

Coping with Anxiety and Depression
SHIRLEY TRICKETT

Coping with Chronic Fatigue
TRUDIE CHALDER

Coping with Depression and Elation
DR PATRICK McKEON

Coping with Fibroids
MARY-CLAIRE MASON

Coping with Rheumatism and Arthritis
DR ROBERT YOUNGSON

Coping with Thyroid Problems
DR JOAN GOMEZ

Curing Arthritis
More ways to a drug-free life
MARGARET HILLS

Curing Arthritis Diet Book
MARGARET HILLS

Curing Arthritis – The Drug-Free Way
MARGARET HILLS

Curing Arthritis Exercise Book
MARGARET HILLS AND JANET HORWOOD

The Good Stress Guide
MARY HARTLEY

Helping Children Cope with Attention Deficit Disorder
DR PATRICIA GILBERT

Helping Children Cope with Divorce
ROSEMARY WELLS

Helping Children Cope with Dyslexia
SALLY RAYMOND

Helping Children Cope with Grief
ROSEMARY WELLS

How to Cope with Difficult People
ALAN HOUEL WITH CHRISTIAN GODEFROY

How to Improve Your Confidence
DR KENNETH HAMBLY

How to Keep Your Cholesterol in Check
DR ROBERT POVEY

How to Start a Conversation and Make Friends
DON GABOR

How to Stick to a Diet
DEBORAH STEINBERG AND DR WINDY DRYDEN

How to Succeed as a Single Parent
CAROLE BALDOCK

The Irritable Bowel Diet Book
ROSEMARY NICOL

The Irritable Bowel Stress Book
ROSEMARY NICOL

Motor Neurone Disease – A Family Affair
DR DAVID OLIVER

The Stress Workbook
JOANNA GUTMANN

The Subfertility Handbook
VIRGINIA IRONSIDE AND SARAH BIGGS

Ten Steps to Positive Living
DR WINDY DRYDEN

Understanding Your Personality
Myers-Briggs and more
PATRICIA HEDGES

Overcoming Common Problems

Coping with Gallstones

Joan Gomez

sheldon **PRESS**

Published in Great Britain in 2000 by
Sheldon Press,
Holy Trinity Church
Marylebone Road
London NW1 4DU

British Library Cataloguing-in-Publication Data

A catalogue record for this book is available
from the British Library

ISBN 0–85969–837–8 ✓

Typeset by Deltatype Limited, Birkenhead, Merseyside
Printed in Great Britain by
Biddles Ltd, Guildford and King's Lynn

Contents

Introduction

My grandmother's gallstone in a bottle on the mantelpiece fascinated all us children, and we often heard the dramatic story of her 'attack of gallstones' – inflammation of the gallbladder, which is another blind alley like the appendix. Rather like acute appendicitis, my grandmother's acute cholecystitis came on out of the blue – probably set off by a stone causing irritation or blockage.

My Great Aunt Mildred, never to be outdone by her sister, suffered from 'gallstone dyspepsia'. She couldn't touch fatty foods, had terrible wind (up and down) and frequent discomfort after meals. Someone had mentioned gallstone dyspepsia and she had latched onto that as the cause of her symptoms. But although modern gastroenterologists – specialists in the digestive system – recognize my aunt's syndrome as common, they are quite certain it is not due to gallstones. That is not to say that gallstones are not prevalent. It is estimated that one person in five, worldwide, has them, with a preponderance in Europe, North America and Australia. Scandinavia comes top of the league in Europe.

The Pima Indians are something special. No one knows how or when they arrived in the brain-baking heat of the Arizona desert, but in centuries past they lived along the banks of the Gila River and called themselves the River People, irrigating their crops by canals. Then, in the late 1880s, along came the Europeans, settled upstream from the Indians and diverted the water supply for their own purposes. The Pimas were left to starve in the arid desert. They moved to the outskirts of the city of Phoenix and in 1963 an epidemic of diabetes – the adult type – swept through their community, thought to be related to their mothers' starvation while they were carrying them.

Now the Pimans are obese, in sedentary work and eating a Western diet. Fifty per cent of them are diabetic and a massive 80 per cent have gallstones with symptoms. It seems that a major disturbance of their digestive metabolism occurred during the famine affecting those close neighbours, the pancreas and the gallbladder. Some researchers believe that the genes are involved, but diet and lifestyle clearly have an effect.

A large number of those of us in the West who are over 40 have gallstones, but most of us are unaware of them, because we have no symptoms. These are called 'silent' gallstones. They are often discovered by accident, for instance if you have an X-ray or an ultrasound examination of your abdomen for something quite unrelated. Surgeons doing an abdominal operation, for example to remove the appendix, check the gallbladder as a matter of routine, and may find stones. The ultimate is when a diagnosis of gallstones is made for the first time at a postmortem, when the patient has lived their whole life without ever knowing they had them. However, even if 80 per cent of gallstones are 'silent', that leaves 20 per cent which cause trouble, while they all have the potential to do so. This is why it is important to know about them, even if you have no gallstone symptoms at present.

How lucky to live now, at the dawn of the second millennium, with a century of medical wonders behind us. When my grandmother and my great aunt had their illnesses the standard remedy for everything was purgation, especially with castor oil, followed by effervescing sodium bicarbonate and (dilute) hydrochloric acid or a mixture of turpentine and ether.

Now we can very safely remove the gallbladder, stones and all, through a keyhole incision, or dispose of some stones *in situ* by dissolving them or breaking them up by harmless, painless electric shocks, given through the skin. New, powerful drugs are being developed all the time and the next improvement in the management of gallstones is most likely to come from the great pharmaceutical industry. The future is full of hope.

Part I
The problems

1

How the gallbladder works

Gall is the old name for bile; it also means bitterness, physical or mental, and is linked in the Bible and Shakespeare with wormwood, a herb with a horrible, acerbic taste. Gallstones are solid lumps of material, formed in the gallbladder from the constituents of bile, so we need to know about bile – where it comes from and what it does.

The liver

The liver is the largest and most important gland in the body, discreetly tucked under the ribcage on the right side of the abdomen. It is a busy chemical factory, underpinning your whole metabolism. It is here that your food is converted into a usable form – you cannot fuel your muscles directly with a bath bun, nor run your brain on fish and chips straight from the plate. Your liver also synthesizes proteins, detoxifies drugs and poisons, and deals with out-dated red blood corpuscles. These are regularly replaced every fortnight or so, and one of their breakdown products is *bilirubin* – 'bili' to do with bile and 'rubin' meaning red, since it is derived from the red pigment in blood. There is also a smaller amount of a greenish pigment, *biliverdin*. If during a stomach upset you bring up some bile you will notice that it is a slightly greeny yellow. Making bile is one of the vital jobs performed by the liver.

Bile

Bile is a sticky yellowish liquid, manufactured continuously, day and night, by the hepatocytes (liver cells) at the rate of half to one litre over the 24 hours. Eating a meal revs up the rate of production – the trigger is a gut hormone called cholecystokinin (cck).

Apart from bilirubin, bile contains cholesterol and some other fats, a little protein and, most importantly, a watery solution of bile salts. These are derived from particular chemicals in blood plasma. They are so precious to the body that they are clawed back from the digested food and bile, in the lowest part of the small intestine, the ileum, and recycled (see Figure 1.1).

Their big task is to make fatty foods digestible, and to make it

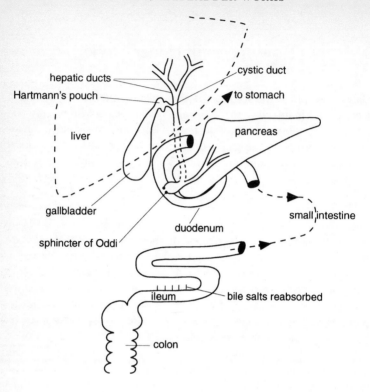

Figure 1 The gallbladder and the bile ducts

possible for the fat-soluble vitamins A, D and K to be absorbed. Fats are broken down with the help of bile into tiny globules of cholesterol, a fact first observed 150 years ago by Rudolf Virchow, a whiz with the then new technology of the microscope. It was this fact that made film star Marilyn Monroe decide to have her healthy gallbladder removed. She reckoned that without it she would be unable to digest fats – and automatically remain slim. Unfortunately for her it does not work like that – as anyone who has had a gallbladder operation for a medical reason will confirm.

Another useful property of bile is the neutralization of the acid from the stomach. It also carries away waste products from the liver 'factory' and is incorporated into the part-digested food products travelling down the intestines. Finally it is bile pigment, derived like the colour of bile itself from blood pigments, which makes the motions yellowy-brown.

The gallbladder

Anatomy

The gallbladder is a little bag containing bile which lies snugly against the liver in the upper right abdomen, hiding behind the duodenum, the part of the intestines leading out of the stomach. It is next to the pancreas. The gallbladder is pear-shaped, 6–8 cm long and 2 or 3 cm across and has a small bulge in its neck, Hartmann's pouch, which is important as a trap for stones – Hartmann was a nineteenth-century anatomist. The gallbladder can hold up to 50 ml of bile, although the normal load is 30 ml (1 fl. oz). Cells in the neck produce mucin or mucus, the whitish glutinous substance the body uses to lubricate tubes and narrow places, for instance the nasal passages. Inflammation or irritation, for example by a gallstone, stimulates mucin production. The *cystic duct*, a small tube 3 or 4 cm long, provides the only way in or out of the gallbladder. It receives an input of bile from the liver by the common hepatic duct, and empties itself as required into the common bile duct. This in turn releases the bile into the duodenum, close to the tube from the pancreas.

A ring of muscle called the *sphincter of Oddi*, after another nineteenth-century Italian physician, controls this outlet. It is usually closed.

Development

The whole liver–gallbladder set-up is so fundamental to life that it begins to form as soon as possible. The liver shows up as an outgrowth from the primitive gut within three weeks of conception, and the foetal liver cells are merrily making bile from the third month. If you are lucky – in about 40 per cent of babies-in-the-making – you can make out the tiny gallbladder itself in the ultrasound film around week 20.

Naturally enough, just as we all differ in the details of such obvious features as our eyes and noses, there can be slight developmental variations in the little tubes around the gallbladder. Some anomalies produce an odd twist or corner where the flow of bile is slowed down or a stone can get caught up. Occasionally someone has a double, or even triple gallbladder, or it may be on the left instead of the right.

7

Madge

Madge was 52 when she was woken up without warning by an intense pain high up on the left side of her abdomen. It would not let up with the homely remedies of a hot water bottle and an indigestion tablet, so she called the emergency doctor. He pointed out that the pain was on the wrong side for the appendix and although she had eaten a rather rich supper it was too severe and unremitting for simple dyspepsia, so he sent her to the local Accident and Emergency department.

Tests and investigations (see Chapter 7) suggested a trapped gallstone and showed that Madge had a left-sided gallbladder and an odd arrangement of the bile ducts, with a stone wedged in one of them. It was decided to remove her gallbladder, since it would be susceptible to further trouble. Although Madge was by no means old, she had a chronic chest disorder, sarcoid, which influenced the surgeon's choice of a keyhole operation rather than open surgery. It means less of a scar and quicker healing, so she was able to go home a few days later.

Physiology: how the gallbladder works

The gallbladder's main tasks are to concentrate the bile which comes fresh from the liver, to store it until it is needed, and to discharge it when a meal arrives in the duodenum. The gallbladder is not just a simple container. Its walls include a layer of smooth muscle, the kind that is controlled by the autonomic (or automatic) nerves. Its major job is to deliver to the duodenum the correct dose of concentrated bile at the appropriate time.

The message to contract, and squeeze out its contents, is conveyed to the gallbladder in two ways: electrically via the nerves, and through the hormone, cck. This is produced to order in the duodenum when food arrives there for the next stage of digestion. The hormone and the nerves operate synergistically – that is, their effect is more than doubled when both act together. Cck also reminds the liver cells to rev up the supply of bile, since it is this which provides the driving force behind the bile in its journey through the gallbladder and the various ducts to the duodenum. The gallbladder also has a hotline to the sphincter of Oddi, the doorway to the duodenum, and conveys when it should relax and let the bile flow through.

To get an idea of the time scale: the gallbladder is exactly halfway through emptying itself just 15 minutes after you have swallowed some liquid nourishment. This has less effect than a meal with solids but is not delayed in the stomach for digestion. The basic stimulus to the gallbladder to contract, and to the sphincter of Oddi to relax, is food entering the digestive system, especially a fatty meal, say bacon, egg, sausage and chips or nut-roast and French fries.

In the *interdigestive period* – the classy term for the time between meals – the gallbladder is relaxed and bile flows into it, while the sphincter of Oddi shuts the system off from the rest of the digestive tract. However, the gallbladder does not lie idle when it is re-loaded. At regular intervals of between one and two hours, a wave of muscular contraction sweeps down the whole of the intestinal tract, and this activity includes the gallbladder. It pushes out about one-third of its contents into the duodenum with each wave.

Processing

The bile is altered or processed in the gallbladder. It loses 75 per cent of its water content for starters, making gallbladder bile between four and ten times more concentrated than liver bile. This makes it more effective as a digestive agent. The down-side is that because it is thicker and even gluey, it is more liable to go lumpy in places – in fact to make gallstones. Apart from being more concentrated, gallbladder bile also differs from liver bile in the proportions of the various constituents (see Table 1.1).

Table 1 Comparison of constituents of liver and the gallbladder

	Liver	Gallbladder
Cholesterol	0.3–3 mmol/l	0.1–87.1 mmol/l
(raw material of cholesterol gallstones)		
Other fats	0.1–2.9 mmol/l	0.1–55.4 mmol/l
Bile salts	0.8–38.1 mmol/l	47.9–275.4 mmol/l
(these are so precious that they are reabsorbed in the small intestine)		
Calcium	10 units	46 units
(extra calcium makes some gallstones show up in an X-ray)		

Pigment: The bile leaving the gallbladder in the common bile duct contains 5 to 10 times as much pigment as the bile coming from the liver.

Lithogenic, that is stone-making, bile means that it is particularly likely to produce gallstones. This occurs if the circulation of bile salts in the liver is slowed down – from problems in the liver itself, such as cirrhosis or hepatitis. A vicious circle develops, with sticky bile leading to sludge and stone formation, in turn increasing the risk of blockage and more stones.

We are not normally aware of the routine physiological activity of our gallbladder any more than of the rest of the normal digestive process – and it is certainly not painful. Pain only crops up in particular circumstances, basically obstruction or infection, or rarely, a tumour. A stone which may have been lying in the gallbladder for months or even years can get stuck in one of the ducts, causing obstruction which the gallbladder muscle struggles – painfully – to overcome. Or an infection may set in especially if the contents of the gallbladder become stagnant, from blockage or other causes.

Problems which are unconnected with gallstones or the gallbladder itself, may confuse the issue, for example, disorders of the chest, back or pancreas. Luckily there are excellent methods for finding the correct diagnosis (Chapter 7), and if necessary, a range of treatments (Chapters 8 and 9).

2

How and why we get gallstones

Not all animals produce gallstones. We share this propensity with our special friends: cats, dogs, horses and cows, while rats do not even have a gallbladder. In humans gallstones affect all races, but some much more than others (see Table 2.1).

Table 2 League table of gallstone sufferers

Nationality	%
Pima Indians in Arizona	80
Chilean Indians	65
Mexican-American women	44
Germany	45
United Kingdom	27
India	20
Italy	20
Denmark	19
Africa	14
Japan	10
China	5

It is estimated that there are 15 to 20 million people in the USA who have gallstones, and 5 to 7 million in the UK.

There are two main types of gallstone: cholesterol and pigment. They differ in appearance, causes, constituents, which treatment works best, in which countries they are found most often – and how they are produced. *Cholesterol stones* are yellowy-white and consist almost entirely of cholesterol – 60 per cent is a minimum. They are far the commonest variety, accounting for three-quarters of the total. They occur mainly in Western cultures, from the UK to the US, from Australia to Sweden – where they are particularly prevalent. They run in families, so that if you have one first-degree blood relative with gallstones your chances of developing them are doubled, with more than one they increase fivefold. Heredity is clearly important, but the cause cannot be only in the genes since immigrants from Africa or Asia who settle in the West develop much the same propensity for cholesterol gallstones as the local population. Also, you run no extra risk if your partner or an adoptive parent has gallstones.

Pigment stones come in black or brown varieties which are quite distinct from each other. Brown pigment stones are found most frequently in the Far East, and account for more than 90 per cent throughout Asia. Pigment stones contain several other constituents as well as pigment, mucus and cholesterol.

How cholesterol stones develop

There are three basic requirements for these stones to form:

1 Excess of cholesterol in the bile, *cholesterolosis*. This can happen with vegetarians as well as meat-eaters – we manufacture our own cholesterol in the liver, from various foods as well as animal fats.
2 Excess of mucin, the slimey material which is designed to protect the lining of the gallbladder from concentrated bile salts. Extra mucin facilitates the formation of crystals of cholesterol and various calcium salts – a basis from which stones easily develop. It is the amount of calcium in a stone which makes it stand out in an X-ray, and black pigment stones seldom have enough.
3 The 'stagnant pool' syndrome (*stasis* or *cholestasis*). There is a sluggish flow of bile and the gallbladder muscle is not emptying it efficiently. This may be due to small, infrequent meals, containing very little fat, such as slimmers and anorexics take, drugs such as pain-killers and tranquillizers which calm down the digestive system and have the side-effect of constipation, or a liver disorder. Another factor is a relative shortage of bile salts, which may be down to failure of cck to stimulate the liver cells sufficiently. This has a knock-on effect, leading to lithogenic bile (see p. 10) with a reduced flow – a vicious circle involving stasis.

Biliary sludge is a semi-liquid like the mud that builds up at the bottom of a pond but not in the bed of a fast-flowing stream. It forms when there is a high cholesterol content in the bile, excess of mucin – and stasis. It is the perfect soil for stones to develop.

Risk factors for cholesterol stones

- Race and family history (see above).
- Increasing age.
- Female sex, especially under forty, but in the elderly the sexes are affected equally.
- Pregnancy: there is a slow-down in the flow of bile and often a resulting build-up of sludge during pregnancy, so that by the time the baby is born 50 per cent of mothers have biliary sludge and 15 per cent have gallstones. The increase in female hormones is responsible. Oestrogen levels are raised throughout pregnancy, plus progesterone in the last three months. By about 12 months after the birth the sludge may have dispersed, but stones are more likely to persist.
- Motherhood – more kids, more stones – each pregnancy increases the risk.
- Malfunction of the gallbladder, so that it does not empty itself effectively or completely. This can be an hereditary fault, in the same way that some of us are better at muscular sports than others.
- Anatomical quirks, individual differences in the geography of the gallbladder or the bile ducts, may impede the flow, as in the case of Madge (see p. 8).
- Excess oestrogen, either naturally as in pregnancy, or through medicines, usually the contraceptive pill or HRT, but also when it is used to treat prostate cancer in men.
- Other medicines, particularly clofibrate (Atromid). This is given to reduce the fat level in the blood, but it boosts the likelihood of gallstones because it floods the bile with the cholesterol it is trying to get rid of. Chlorpromazine (Largactil) and other major tranquillizers also increase the risk of gallstones.
- Being overweight – this may be quite moderate, and it seems that it is a generous intake of food rather than the degree of actual fatness which counts.
- Rapid weight loss, especially based on a very low fat diet, kills the production of cck, the vital stimulus to the production of bile salts and the emptying of the gallbladder. Complete fasts, and very long-term low calorie diets have the same effect. This seems so unfair, since the overweight people who abound in the West are extra susceptible to gallstones and are frequently advised to diet.
- Diet in relation to gallstones is confusing. The only certainty is

that refined white sugar increases the risk, as discovered in Australia where sugar-laden soft drinks are very popular. In Chile, where there is a high incidence of stones, they eat a large amount of legumes (vegetables with pods, like beans and peas) – this may be relevant. Although a high fibre, low fat diet would seem sensible, there is absolutely no evidence of its making any difference. The good news is that moderate amounts of alcohol have no adverse effect on stone formation, while coffee is definitely beneficial. Smoking, as with most health issues, makes matters worse.

- Some unrelated illnesses increase the likelihood of cholesterol gallstones. They include cirrhosis, chronic hepatitis, tumour and other long-term liver disorders; cystic fibrosis; diabetes; and the aftermath of operations on the stomach. However, uncomplicated Crohn's disease does not increase the risk for this type of gallstone, as was formerly believed.

Angela

It all started when her doctor suggested she should lose some weight for the sake of her health. He even pointed out that she was a likely candidate for gallstones because she had the five 'F's which traditionally are said to favour them. She was:

- fair – a honey blonde;
- fat – 11 stone 8 lbs at 5 ft 3 ins (66.6 kg at 1.6 m);
- fertile – she had three lovely children;
- forty – she was 44;
- and finally she was female.

The doctor did not expect her to act on his advice so promptly and efficiently and so he did not warn her to aim at gradual weight reduction, say 1–2 lbs or 0.45–0.9 kg a week. But Angela made an all-out effort, partly to encourage Brian, her husband. His blood pressure was going up in line with his weight – he had been piling it on ever since he gave up playing football. Every evening they went either to the pool or the gym, but more importantly all fats were deleted from their diet together with almost everything sweet. Life was no fun, but it worked – for Brian.

Angela was proud to have peeled off nearly a stone in the first three weeks. She felt good – lighter, but a little tired, and she had one or two short-lived twinges of abdominal pain. She felt that they both deserved one decent meal to celebrate their success.

They did not go over the top – just a pizza followed by fruit salad and cream, with a glass of white wine. Oddly, Angela did not feel as hungry as she had expected, and what had been a niggling pain suddenly switched on full power. The doctor noticed at once that she was jaundiced, the whites of her eyes tinged yellow.

It turned out that a single large stone had lodged in the common bile duct, producing back pressure on the liver. In the hospital investigations were made at emergency speed, followed by an open operation to remove both gallbladder and stone. Keyhole surgery or an endoscopic procedure (see Chapter 9) might have been used had the need for treatment been less urgent.

How pigment stones develop

My grandmother's cholesterol stone was a dingy yellowish-white. Pigment stones come in two distinct colours – black and brown. They also differ in chemical composition, causation and the way they are formed – and where. The colour in both types comes from bilirubin.

Black pigment stones

Black pigment stones account for nearly 25 per cent of gallstones and are next commonest to cholesterol stones. Like them they affect mainly Western communities and always develop within the gallbladder, in association with an excess of mucin. However, although they contain 20 per cent cholesterol, they are far harder than cholesterol stones, of the same homogeneous consistency throughout, and virtually impossible to dissolve. Because they contain plenty of calcium, 95 per cent of them show up well on X-ray, as do some cholesterol stones. Black stones are prone to lodge in the common bile duct, producing back pressure on the liver and jaundice, particularly if the gallbladder is on the left.

Excess of bilirubin in the bile is the underlying cause of black pigment stones, together with a shortage of bile salts. This can occur in several conditions affecting the blood:

- hereditary blood disorders such as sickle cell disease, spherocytosis and thalassaemia. The more severe the anaemia the greater the likelihood of gallstones;
- cirrhosis of the liver, alcoholic or otherwise: 30 per cent of those with chronic liver disease have black stones;

- 'artificial' heart valves, which tend to damage the red blood corpuscles as they pass through the heart;
- Crohn's disease with a stricture or the after-effects of operations on the small intestine. Any damage or disease of the small intestine can increase the likelihood of these stones;
- feeding intravenously in the course of an illness or operation on the digestive system, so-called *total parenteral nutrition*;
- advancing age increases the risk of black stones, but sex makes no difference.

Acute pancreatitis, inflammation of the pancreas, is a common, severe complication of small black stones, which may block the pancreatic duct.

Brown pigment stones

Brown pigment stones are the least common, accounting for less than 5 per cent of the total. They are found most often in the Orient. In Hong Kong, Korea and South-East Asia an infection of the small ducts within the liver – *pyogenic cholangitis* – is fairly common. The infection can spread to the hepatic ducts, the cystic duct, the gallbladder and the common bile ducts. Particular strains of bacteria release bilirubin from blood cells, or there may be a parasitic infection of the intestines.

Typically, brown stones are formed in the ducts not the gallbladder, from a sludge of mucin and bacteria. The main problem is obstruction, with a vicious circle of infection – blockage – stone formation – blockage – infection . . . Brown stones often form round a small black or cholesterol stone which is causing stasis and an increased risk of infection. As with black stones, neither sex is more susceptible than the other, but age increases the risk. These stones are soft and crumbly and easily broken up or dissolved. They are radiolucent, that is, they do not show up on a plain X-ray but may be detected with ultrasound.

The size of the stones

If conditions favour the development of gallstones of any of the three types, for example, if there is sludge and a poorly contracting gallbladder, it is more likely that existing stones will become larger than that a fresh crop of small stones will appear. The rate of 'growth' is slow: 1–4 mm per year. Obviously one big stone is more likely to cause trouble than several small ones which can be carried away in the bile. A big stone may get stuck in a tiny duct, or it may cause pressure and damage the lining of the gallbladder, causing inflammation: chronic or acute cholecystitis. Finally, a stone may ulcerate through the gallbladder wall, involving another organ and causing serious problems (see pp. 27, 29, 79).

Prevention of gallstones

Cholesterol stones

Since three factors are necessary simultaneously for the development of these stones, correcting any one of these should prevent or halt their formation.

1 Overproduction of cholesterol is checked by taking bile salts: the natural form chenodeoxycholic acid, which may cause diarrhoea, or ursodeoxycholic acid (UDCA) – trade names: Destolit, Ursofalk, Urdox – nightly. Unfortunately they clash with the contraceptive pill and other oestrogen-containing medicines, clofibrate and antacids.
2 Overproduction of mucin is controlled by the non-steroidal anti-inflammatories (NSAIDs) used in arthritis and other painful conditions (Brufen, Feldene, Mobic and others), also aspirin.
3 A lazy gallbladder can be given a kick-start with a derivative of cck, cholecystokinin octapeptide, given into a vein.

Also, keep slim, do not overdo the sweet foods, but do not cut out all fats. Regular balanced meals three times a day make better sense than grazing or snacking through the day, with no definite stimulus to the gallbladder.

Black pigment stones

Have treatment for any blood or liver disorder.

Brown pigment stones

The only ploy is to try to avoid developing either cholesterol or black pigment stones since they often provide the focus for a bunch of bacteria to settle in, and also act as a starting point on which the brown material can build.

Jeff

Jeff was everybody's friend – easy-going, happy-go-lucky, he enjoyed life to the full, including smokes, booze and grub – especially the sweet course. The floor of his car was littered with chocolate wrappers and empty lager cans and the ashtrays were overflowing. He got away with it, apparently unscathed, for 60 years – thanks to an excellent constitution. His lungs and his digestion stood up to his lifestyle without complaint, but at 61 he developed the non-insulin-dependent type of diabetes, like his mother before him. He also began to show signs of alcoholic liver disease, with abdominal pain, an enlarged, tender liver and a hint of jaundice in the whites of his eyes.

Cholestasis was part of the syndrome and he developed chronic inflammation of the gallbladder. At the cholecystectomy operation – removal of the gallbladder – it was found to be full of yellowy-white cholesterol stones and some of the black pigment type. Jeff had to start on anti-diabetic treatment and undertake a complete overhaul of his way of living to set him on the road to survival. He was an intelligent man and discovered new pleasures in golf, music, reading and the Internet. With his outgoing personality he soon made some new, non-drinking friends, and managed to keep his job.

3

Gallstone disorders and biliary colic

Most of us have some gallstones by the time we reach the age of 50. You may have gallstones which remain 'silent' and never give you any trouble. This is what happens in the majority of cases. When you have had gallstones for five years, you only stand a 10 per cent chance of having symptoms, and after 15 to 20 years the risk goes up by a mere 8 per cent. Even if you do develop gallstone symptoms, the outlook is not too bad:

- No one ever dies just from having gallstones.
- It is uncommon for them to cause major problems.
- Most people with a definite gallstone disorder will not need an operation.
- There is a choice of treatments.

Gallstones only make a nuisance of themselves if they get stuck, either in the little pouch near the exit of the gallbladder or in one of the bile ducts nearby. The symptom that should alert you to the possibility of a gallstone disorder is one you cannot ignore – PAIN. The likeliest causes are biliary colic, the commoner, or inflammation of the gallbladder (cholecystitis).

Biliary colic

This is usually set off by partial or intermittent obstruction by a stone and comprises what is familiarly known as 'an attack of gallstones'. The pain is intense and comes on suddenly, often waking the victim from sleep. The term 'colic' is a misnomer. Colicky pain, such as the green apple variety, comes in waves, whereas this pain is continuous. It goes on without let-up for at least 20 minutes and for more than an hour in 60 per cent of cases. If it persists for over six hours it means that a complication has set in, probably inflammation of the gallbladder or its near neighbour, the pancreas.

The position of gallstone pain, the muscle pain from the gallbladder's strong contractions against the obstruction, is important in making the diagnosis. Typically, you feel it in the upper right-hand quadrant of your abdomen and also between your shoulder blades or at the tip of your right shoulder. The latter is called 'referred' pain because although it is felt in one area it refers to another, where the trouble really lies, and which shares the same nerve supply. Variations are pain in the back or neck, on the left instead of the right, or like a band round the lower chest or upper abdomen. Some people suffer from nausea and may vomit, but this is not a particular characteristic of biliary colic, and such symptoms as flatulence, bloating, dyspepsia or bowel upset are definitely not part of it.

Especially if the pain is not felt in the usual site, it can be difficult for your doctor to diagnose its cause. Conditions which can mimic gallstone pain include:

- Heart attack, when the coronary arteries supplying the heart muscle are furred up, or a shorter-lived pain if they go into spasm.
- Pancreatitis – acute or chronic inflammation of the pancreas. The acute type usually follows a big meal with plenty of alcohol: it is very painful and apt to cause mental disturbances including hallucinations. It can be started by a gallstone blocking the pancreatic duct (see below). Chronic pancreatitis, by contrast, is almost always due to too much alcohol, and affects mainly men between 35 and 45.
- Peptic ulcer – sudden severe pain occurs with a perforated ulcer, but there will have been milder ulcer symptoms previously, after meals or when the stomach and duodenum were empty.
- Kidney disease – kidney stone causes excruciating pain, typically in the loin.
- Aneurysm – a split in the wall of the aorta, the main artery running down the middle of the body. The pain is central, too.
- Oesophagitis – inflammation of the gullet, often associated with hiatus hernia.
- Irritable bowel syndrome (IBS) – this is often misdiagnosed as biliary colic, especially the 'hepatic flexure syndrome' when the bowel high up under the liver on the right of the abdomen is in spasm. The pain is in the gallbladder area, but is more likely to be truly colicky, waxing and waning. The give-away symptoms of IBS include bloating of the abdomen, alternating bouts of diarrhoea and constipation and relief after passing a motion. It is a very common disorder, particularly in women.
- Chest disease, for example pleurisy in which the pain is worse if

you take a deep breath, or basal pneumonia in which you are short of breath.

Biliary colic may pass off without treatment – a stone may move on spontaneously – or after one of several methods of alleviating the situation. Unfortunately, although you can have gallstones in your gallbladder for years without any problems, once you have had an attack of biliary colic you are likely to get repeats increasingly frequently.

Glenda

Glenda had typical biliary colic. The first time was just before her sixty-fifth birthday. She and her friend Laura had gone away to a hotel for a few days' break. In the middle of the second night Glenda had a dreadful tummy pain and, to her surprise, a pain at the tip of her right shoulder. It was much worse than the twinges she got from her hiatus hernia. Although she did not vomit, Glenda felt nauseated.

It was awkward being away from home. She did not want to spoil the holiday so she played down how bad she felt. After about half-an-hour the pain began to ease off, but it left Glenda feeling weak and she could not face much food for the rest of their stay. She put the episode down to a nasty bout of indigestion and vowed never again to trust hotel meals. However, when she had a similar attack two months later at home, she had only eaten the plain fare she had prepared herself. She told her doctor about it, and he said to call him at once if it happened a third time.

It did, and again subsided, more or less, over 24 hours. This time the doctor arranged for Glenda to see a gastroenterologist. She had a battery of tests of which the most useful was an ultrasound. Her gallbladder was full of small stones and it was clear that now and again one of them might get into the cystic duct, causing severe pain. There was a constant risk of the gallbladder becoming inflamed. There was no doubt about what to do.

Glenda had her gallbladder removed and with it her recurrent attacks of biliary colic.

Gallstone in the common bile duct: choledocholithiasis

The simplest form of biliary colic occurs when a stone lodges in the neck of the gallbladder or the cystic duct without causing complete blockage, but in 10–15 per cent of cases a stone slips into the common bile duct and sticks there (see Figure 2). Sometimes this does not produce any symptoms, but more often it sets off one of a variety of problems.

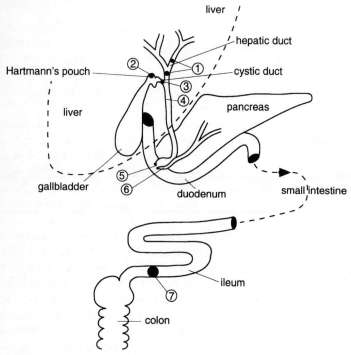

Figure 2 Places where gallstones may stick

Key:
1 One of the hepatic ducts, 2 Hartmann's pouch, 3 Cystic duct, 4 Common bile duct, 5 Sphincter of Oddi, 6 Pancreatic duct, 7 Ileum

Jaundice

Jaundice just means 'yellow' – remember your French, 'jaune'. It refers to a yellowing of the skin. It may be due to an excess of carrots in anorexia nervosa, the anti-malaria drug mepacrine, excessive breakdown of red blood cells in some blood diseases, or a liver disorder. Gallstones can cause *obstructive jaundice*, due to blockage by a stone in the common bile duct or – less commonly – in the common hepatic duct or one of its tributaries. This usually, but not invariably, leads to a build-up of bile pigment in the tissues, giving them the yellowish tinge. It is most noticeable in the whites of the eyes, and you may itch all over. The latter is because of the irritant effect of the bile salts caught up with the pigment. In this situation your motions will be pale – putty-coloured – but your urine orange or extra dark.

Sometimes a stone gets stuck fast in the common bile duct or one of the hepatic ducts when there is a strong flow of bile, but when the flow slackens the bile can get past the stone – a ball-valve effect that can produce jaundice which fluctuates with the shifting of the stone.

A vague, dull ache in your upper abdomen when you have jaundice is caused by the stretching of the capsule – skin – of the liver when it is swollen, for instance with hepatitis. A severe pain with jaundice is likely to be due to a stone passing, or trying to pass, down the common bile duct, but in an elderly person the first warning can be the sudden onset of mental confusion and physical prostration. In a prolonged obstruction in the common bile duct, even if the symptoms seem quite mild, there may be bleeding from varicose veins in the gullet. This may cause a vomit streaked with blood or, more often, looking like coffee grounds, with black motions from altered blood. It can happen when the liver, under back pressure from the blockage is no longer making adequate supplies of the clotting factor, and the same back pressure leads to swollen veins in the oesophagus.

Any of these symptoms can occur even after the gallbladder has been removed, either because a stone has remained in the common bile duct – and probably grown bigger – or a new one has developed.

Edward

Edward was 81, hardly any age nowadays. He was quite fit and played nine holes of golf regularly and was what he called a 'good trencherman'. In his sixties he had been through a bad patch with gallstone trouble, but imagined that he had said goodbye to that forever when he had his cholecystectomy.

His illness took everyone by surprise. With no more warning than 24 hours off his food, he startled his wife by asking her if they had met before and what he was doing in this place. He looked ill and lay on his bed until the GP came and swept him off to hospital. Physical examination, X-rays and ultrasound, and blood tests showing a very high level of bilirubin and other chemicals, gave clues to the situation – stone in the common bile duct. In view of his age it was decided to avoid open operation and the stone was removed by an endoscopic manoeuvre (see pp. 61, 68).

Acute cholangitis

Acute cholangitis (the Western variety) means inflammation of the bile passages within the liver due to a cholesterol or black pigment stone made in the gallbladder travelling down the cystic duct, then backwards towards the liver, becoming impacted in a hepatic duct. Although no infection is involved initially, unlike the situation in the oriental type of cholangitis, bacteria sneak in secondarily in 90 per cent of cases.

Recurrent pyogenic cholangitis

Recurrent pyogenic cholangitis (pyogenic means there is pus) is common in Hong Kong, Korea and all of South-East Asia. The first event is an infection which causes the cholangitis. The culprit is often a strain of E.coli, or a parasite. These organisms form the basis of brown pigment stones in the bile ducts. Usually there is a period of malaise and mild abdominal discomfort followed by repeated attacks of acute illness, with jaundice and pale motions, when a stone or stones cause a blockage.

Pancreatitis

A gallstone in the common bile duct may also block the duct from the pancreas, which usually shares the exit into the duodenum through the sphincter of Oddi (see Figure 1.1). One in 12 gallstone sufferers will develop acute pancreatitis at some time, and this rises to one in four if the stones are small. The symptoms are like those of biliary colic, but worse if the condition is acute, and milder but recurrent, if it is chronic. In an acute phase there is a sudden rush of intense pain high in the abdomen with nausea and vomiting. Quite frequently the unfortunate sufferer develops both acute pancreatitis and acute gallbladder disease, cholecystitis, at the same time, while in one in five cases of acute pancreatitis there is also acute cholangitis.

It is not all doom and gloom, however. Most gallstones which block the pancreatic duct do so only temporarily, and are passed out into the duodenum which is close at hand. Only a large stone can cause a hold-up in the wider tubing of a normal intestine, and the type most likely to cause trouble are the brown pigment stones which develop outside the gallbladder.

Gallstone in the intestine

It is a rare occurrence for a stone to cause obstruction in the much wider tubing of the intestines. This is only likely to happen when there is a diseased segment of the small intestine which is abnormally narrowed, as in Crohn's disease. Recurrent attacks of colic due to obstruction are common in this disorder, apart from gallstones.

Gallstones and cancer

Cancer of the gallbladder is the only kind associated with gallstones, but it is very rare, and on the decrease in the West. The risk factors are extra large stones and a large amount of calcium in the wall of the gallbladder. Both of these will show up in an ordinary X-ray or with ultrasound, giving you and your doctor plenty of warning of a possible danger – which can be abolished by removing the gallbladder.

4

Cholecystitis

Inflammation of the gallbladder – cholecystitis – may be acute or it may be chronic.

Acute cholecystitis

Acute inflammation of the gallbladder is almost always caused by a stone lodging in Hartmann's pouch or in the small cystic duct. Just occasionally the gallbladder may be blocked off by a wodge of thick mucus, a worm or – rarely – a tumour. The inflammation goes through two phases:

1 *Chemical* – irritation from the concentrated bile salts trapped in the gallbladder instead of being emptied out into the duodenum after every meal.
2 *Bacterial* – in half of those whose gallbladder is cut off in this way an infection starts up in the stagnant bile, worsening the inflammation and making it more dangerous.

Prompt treatment may 'catch' the illness before it has developed into the second stage.

In 10 per cent of those with all the features of inflammation of the gallbladder there is a conundrum. The symptoms are indistinguishable from inflammation due to a blockage, but there is no stone or other obstruction to be found. This situation has an impressive name: *acalculous cholecystitis* (see p. 31).

The cardinal features of acute cholecystitis are those of biliary colic, including right upper abdominal pain radiating to the right shoulder or between the shoulder blades, plus these extra signs and symptoms:

- restlessness;
- sweating;
- vomiting;
- pale skin;
- fever, sometimes with rigors (shivering attacks in which you feel deadly cold, although you are burning hot);

- fast pulse;
- involuntary tensing up of your abdominal muscles when you breathe in – your doctor can feel this: it is called Murphy's sign;
- similarly, a tightening of the muscles in response to light pressure in the upper right part of the abdomen – a protective reflex called guarding;
- tenderness to pressure over the area;
- swelling of the skin there, which gives to pressure like the oedema of swollen ankles;
- jaundice.

Of course, you will not have every one of these nasties, for instance you have only a one in four risk of jaundice, but these are the things to look out for.

Conditions which may resemble acute cholecystitis
- all those mentioned in connection with biliary colic (see p. 19);
- appendicitis, particularly if the appendix is tucked behind the first part of the colon (retrocaecal appendicitis);
- epidemic myalgia – pain in the muscles in a localized area;
- shingles – a rash follows the pain;
- porphyria: a disease which includes attacks of acute abdominal pain and psychiatric upset;
- STD – sexually transmitted disease – an infection with gonorrhoea or chlamydia can spread from the vagina to cause biliary symptoms.

Sometimes acute inflammation of the gallbladder will subside without your taking any action, but it is certain to come back. On the other hand, without treatment the disease may progress disastrously to empyema, a gallbladder full of pus, which occurs in up to 11 per cent of cases. Or a stone may perforate the gallbladder wall and set off peritonitis, a dangerous infection of the membranes clothing the abdominal organs; or it may form a false passage, a fistula, into the intestine.

Elderly people are very much at risk, although their symptoms may not be as dramatic as in a younger person. In an old person any symptoms suggesting cholecystitis must be taken seriously and anyone with diabetes is especially vulnerable. They tend to have rather large, inefficient gallbladders which do not fill properly and contract only weakly and irregularly. This may not matter much in the ordinary way, but if a diabetic develops cholecystitis he or she is likely to do badly, with a particular propensity for the gallbladder to fill with pus. Surgery is essential, although it is more than usually likely to run into complications.

If you are a sufferer in the senior years, or have diabetes, even if your symptoms do not seem all that severe, or they let up from time to time, do not be lulled into being brave or 'not making a fuss'. See your doctor as an emergency, not by one of those appointments booked many days ahead. Better safe than sorry.

The important treatments – emergency, immediate, follow-on and long-term – are outlined on p. 73.

Enid

Enid was a healthy 78-year-old when she developed all the symptoms to suggest acute cholecystitis – pain, nausea, vomiting, and a raised temperature, and she looked dreadfully ill. She was one of the 25 per cent who develop jaundice. The doctor was not sure whether he could feel a swollen gallbladder under Enid's ribs on the right, but the place was too tender for him to press hard. Blood tests indicated a severe infection – she had a very high white cell count, and ultrasound showed stones in the gallbladder area. It was decided to operate. The gallbladder was found to be full of pus – 50 per cent of empyema cases are not diagnosed before surgery. After the removal of her gallbladder under an umbrella of antibiotics, Enid recovered slowly but steadily, although it took five weeks for her skin to lose its yellow tint.

Acute emphysematous cholecystitis

This is an unpleasant and serious form of cholecystitis. Elderly men with diabetes are particularly susceptible. It comes on with acute pain, shock and rapid general physical deterioration. It is a dangerous condition, caused by gas-forming bacteria infecting the gallbladder. In an X-ray film the gas shows up as dark areas in the gallbladder and its ducts. Surgery is needed urgently and can be life-saving.

Secondary complications of acute cholecystitis

These three are highly dangerous:

- liver abscess;
- empyema – pus – in the chest;
- septicaemia – the infection has got into the bloodstream.

In contrast to appendicitis, there is one serious complication that hardly ever arises in cholecystitis – perforation or bursting of the inflamed organ, causing the abdominal disaster of general peritonitis. The wall of the gallbladder is full of muscle, and inflammation tends to make it all the thicker.

Chronic cholecystitis

This is very different from acute cholecystitis, and a troublesome disease in its own right. It nearly always recurs after a heavy meal. It may be caused by gallstones irritating or intermittently blocking the gallbladder, or to super-concentrated, irritating bile, and/or an infection. The wall of the gallbladder becomes thickened and stiff with fibrous scar tissue and overworked muscle. Sometimes there are little bulges between the bundles of muscles fibres and these trap bacteria to form focuses of infection: Rokitansky-Aschoff sinuses – a sinus is a dead end. There are likely to be ulcers in the mucous lining of the gallbladder, and a mucocoele may form, that is a blister of mucus, if the outlet from the gallbladder is restricted while it is still producing mucus. Sometimes the whole gallbladder may fill with mucus (hydrops). The cystic duct may become occluded by scar tissue or more often a stone, putting pressure on the gallbladder muscle to contract, worsening the situation.

How chronic cholecystitis shows up

- biliary colic symptoms;
- nausea usually;
- vomiting often, but later in the illness;
- attacks of pain following a heavy meal or a fatty snack;
- sudden pain behind the breastbone, raising the question of heart attack (an electrocardiogram is an essential check);
- sweating *without any fever*;
- fast pulse;
- tenderness in the upper right-hand quarter of the abdomen;
- sleeping in the prone position may cause pain because it increases the likelihood of a stone getting into the cystic duct.

Complications

- acute cholecystitis;
- fistula – a false passage from the gallbladder into another organ;
- sinuses – cul-de-sacs of infection;

- gangrene of the gallbladder, if the blood supply is impeded;
- gallstone ileus – paralysis of the intestines: an emergency;
- 'porcelain gallbladder' – deposits of calcium in the wall of the gallbladder, which cannot then function;
- Mirizzi's syndrome – see below;
- cancer of the gallbladder;
- the life-threatening secondary complications of acute cholecystitis (see above).

All of these, except the first, are rare. Ultrasound with computerized tomography (CT) scanning if necessary, will pinpoint the site of the problem in most cases.

Peter

Peter was in his fifties and worked in a city firm. He believed he had an ulcer, or at least troublesome indigestion, for which he took some white medicine. It did not help much. His job involved a number of sumptuous dinners with clients, but he was careful not to overdo the wine and he never touched brandy or spirits. It was the sweets he could not resist – delicious desserts, smothered in cream or cream-ice.

He would be woken – if he got as far as bed – by a sharp pain in the top right-hand corner of his abdomen. Usually it had passed off by the morning and each time he swore to eat like a monk with plain fare. When he kept to this he did not have as many attacks, but they certainly did not stop. He then discovered, by a curious chance, one factor that seemed to be relevant. His wife was discussing babies, a favourite subject now they had a new grandson. The baby obstinately refused to sleep on his back, the way they recommend nowadays, but preferred to lie on his tummy. 'Like me,' said Peter. Then he began to notice that he often had an attack when he slept front down.

He was not crazy. In this position there is a tendency for any stone in the gallbladder to slip down into the cystic duct where it will cause pain, even if it moves into the common bile duct later. Investigations showed that Peter had numerous stones in his gallbladder and that its wall was unduly thick and inflexible. It was an unhealthy organ, which could no longer work effectively. The best and safest course was to get rid of it surgically, and into the bargain avoid the risk of unpleasant and dangerous complications.

Mirizzi's syndrome

This is one of the complications that Peter side-stepped. Sometimes the gallbladder is bulging with stones and presses on the common bile duct, blocking it from outside. The results are similar to those of the more usual blockage from a stone inside the duct, with jaundice the most obvious effect (see p. 22). In Mirizzi's syndrome a stone in the gallbladder erodes its way through into the common bile duct (*cholecystocholedochal fistula* – try impressing your friends with that!) Treatment is one of several sophisticated surgical manoeuvres (see Chapter 9).

Acalculous cholecystitis

This type of cholecystitis, characterized by the absence of gallstones, comes in both acute and chronic forms.

Acute acalculous cholecystitis

The symptoms are indistinguishable from those of severe, acute inflammation of the gallbladder, and it arises in 10 per cent of cases presenting as such. It is on the increase. Stones or not, there is no way that this illness is 'all in the mind'. It is as genuine and serious as the type it resembles, and is more fraught with dangers, for example of severe bacterial infection, empyema, gangrene or perforation. The underlying problem is often *ischaemia* of the gallbladder, an impaired blood supply due to the furred arteries of atherosclerosis, high blood pressure or vasculitis – inflamed blood vessels.

Chronic acalculous cholecystitis

The symptoms are those of mild biliary colic, and investigations show that the filling and emptying of the gallbladder are faulty and irregular. Another characteristic is *microlithiasis* – numerous crystals of cholesterol, rather than fewer but larger stones. These can be seen by X-ray, and the distended state of the gallbladder and bile ducts can be picked up with ultrasound.

Although in half the cases, acalculous cholecystitis appears without any hint of where it has come from, there are a number of conditions which may be associated with it:

- specific infections, such as typhoid fever;

31

- heart failure;
- serious physical trauma or major surgery;
- metabolic disturbances such as diabetes, alcoholism, pernicious anaemia;
- rheumatoid arthritis, lupus, polyarteritis, Crohn's disease.

Treatment must embrace any underlying or associated disorder, but most sufferers are vastly improved by having their gallbladders removed, although they contain no stones.

The post-cholecystectomy syndrome

Usually, removing the gallbladder should mean a happy ending to gallstone problems. You only stand a 5 per cent risk of serious after-effects from the operation, although 40 per cent of patients have some symptoms. Most people with the syndrome feel that all their original symptoms are coming back – whether these amounted to mild or full-blown biliary colic. This is a puzzle.

Either the symptoms had been due to something other than gallbladder disease in the first place; or the operation itself has damaged the bile duct system; or third, a totally unrelated disorder has cropped up, which is mistakenly interpreted as a return of the previous trouble. There are three main types of post-cholecystectomy syndrome:

- physical: jaundice, if it occurs, always indicates a physical problem;
- faulty functioning of the digestive or biliary system without any disease;
- psychosomatic – usually mediated through stress, depression or anxiety.

Important causes include:

- bile duct stones which had not been removed at the operation or have developed since (30 per cent);
- mistiming of the sphincter of Oddi (9 per cent);
- peptic ulcer (5 per cent);
- tumour in the area of the pancreas, liver or gallbladder;
- chronic pancreatitis;

- stricture – narrowing of one of the bile ducts by scarring that has resulted from damage by a stone and/or infection;
- irritable bowel;
- hiatus hernia, inflammation of the gullet;
- flatulent dyspepsia;
- hepatitis – even painful back problems may produce confusing symptoms.

Sharon

Sharon had several bouts of biliary colic in her forties, but it was not until she was 50 that she had the big one. She would never forget it. It was during her honeymoon. The marriage was the second time round for both of them, and because money was tight they had chosen a holiday walking in the Lakes. After a long day of fresh air and exercise they were as hungry as hunters and ate a huge meal of the brunch variety – sausages, bacon, eggs, French fries and baked beans.

Sharon was mildly regretting that she had eaten so much when she was suddenly doubled up in agony. The pain went through from the gallbladder area to a spot between her shoulder blades. She flinched when the doctor pressed gently over the site of the pain in the front, and she found herself sweating. She was not sick. After an injection of pethidine and plenty of fluids Sharon was together enough to give her view on the treatment she wanted for her acute cholecystitis. She chose the standard cholecystec-tomy operation since it is very safe and has a high long-term success rate.

However, Sharon was one of the unlucky ones; but it was not until two years later that her symptoms returned with a vengeance. She had pain in the upper abdomen and was losing weight – without trying. Liver function tests showed normal and there was nothing significant in an ultrasound examination. In the end a CT scan (computerized tomography) revealed one big stone in the common bile duct. This was removed through an endoscope (see pp. 61, 68). Leafing through the old notes it seemed that the bile ducts had not been investigated thoroughly enough at the time of the original operation. One small stone must have been overlooked – and it had grown.

The major lessons for all of us to learn from what happened to other people, like Madge, Peter and Sharon, is that while gallstones may lie doggo for years, once you have experienced a bout of biliary colic, or have discovered accidentally that you have gallstones, you must be super-alert to any upper abdominal pains and take them seriously. Do not delay having treatment – it is never convenient – since if you wait the situation will arise, sooner or later, when there is an emergency and you have little choice about which treatment you would prefer.

5

Biliary dyspepsia

Biliary colic, obstructive jaundice and acute cholecystitis are all symptoms or complications that can confidently be ascribed to gallstones. Another syndrome, equally distressing, is even more common and crops up just as often whether there are gallstones present or not. Biliary dyspepsia, flatulent dyspepsia and gallstone dyspepsia – are all terms that refer to this group of symptoms which are not caused by gallstones! Nevertheless, gallstones are often blamed. It is totally different from acalculous cholecystitis, in which there are the characteristic symptoms of acute or chronic inflammation of the gallbladder (see p. 26).

Biliary dyspepsia affects women twice as often as men, especially between the ages of 20 and 40. Ten to 19 and 60 to 69 are the most vulnerable periods for men, although no age is exempt. The symptoms are a variable bunch, but you will not have them all:

- vague pain or discomfort roughly in the upper right-hand quarter of your abdomen, the gallbladder area, but sometimes on the left or all over;
- intolerance of fatty foods, causing pain, vomiting, headache or diarrhoea;
- regurgitation of food, and heartburn;
- loss of appetite, although this is not general and there is seldom any weight loss;
- nausea and in some cases, vomiting;
- feeling full halfway through the meal;
- bloating – distension after a few mouthfuls of food or drink, or as the day wears on;
- burping, belching and, less often, farting;
- unpleasant taste in the mouth;
- waterbrash – saliva suddenly fills your mouth, a reflex from some irritation in the digestive system;
- bowel disturbance;
- headache, fatigue, feeling generally unwell (malaise).

The pain or discomfort may be better or worse after food, or unaffected and passing a motion does not usually relieve it.

The causes of this type of dyspepsia can include:

- serious physical problems, such as Crohn's disease, cystic fibrosis, pancreatic disorders, heart, kidney or liver failures, cancers anywhere, e.g. the lung;
- medication – anti-inflammatories (NSAIDs), digoxin, antibiotics, analgesics;
- pregnancy;
- oesophagitis – inflammation of the gullet, often alcoholic;
- hiatus hernia;
- cigarettes;
- alcohol in excess;
- depression or anxiety due to a stressful life-event or a chronic worry;
- a physical stress such as a bout of flu or a rigorous slimming campaign can also trigger the disorder.

There will be other indications of what is wrong in these cases. If none of them fits the bill you are left with what is called *functional dyspepsia*. 'Functional' means that no physical cause can be found, but this is not to say that the symptoms are not wretched and upsetting.

Functional dyspepsia can be distinguished from other types by the following clues:

- the pain occurs every day, starting in the mornings, not in bouts or episodes;
- it may last all day until bedtime, usually unaffected by food (some people are made worse), or indigestion medicines;
- it covers a wide, ill-defined area of your abdomen and may include two separate places;
- it is rare for functional pain to break through your sleep and wake you, although it generally starts up soon after you have woken naturally;
- vomiting brings you no relief and you feel weak and poorly and unable to face any food for several hours afterwards. This contrasts with the situation in ulcer pain in which vomiting leaves you feeling better, so that you are able to eat almost straight away.
- bowel movements, similarly, are no help in biliary dyspepsia.

For older sufferers in particular, say 45-plus, a few investigations are usually made to show up any undiagnosed disorders and pinpoint those that are treatable. The tests include blood tests for general health and the presence of infection, a test on the motions for signs of bleeding anywhere in the digestive tract, a barium meal to outline on X-ray abnormalities in the stomach or duodenum, an endoscopy to check the stomach and oesophagus lining for inflammation, and liver enzyme tests for alcoholic or other liver disorders.

Maeve

Maeve had half the traditional features of gallstone sufferers. She was blonde and plump – she felt this was partly the appearance from bloating – but she was only 25 years old. She had been having abdominal pain all day and every day, for more than a month. She also found that she could not eat fried foods 'without paying for it' by feeling sick. Her doctor tried her with antacids (Gaviscon), antispasmodics (Colofac), and anti-nausea tablets (Domperidone). With each new prescription she felt a little better – but only for a few days. In the end the GP sent her to the gastroenterology clinic at the hospital. Ultrasound and an examination by endoscopy were carried out, a breath test for helicobacter pylori, the stomach bug, as well as the standard blood tests – all were disappointingly negative.

Although she found chamomile tea quite soothing, none of the herbal medicines from the local health store really helped. Much against her feelings, she was persuaded to talk things through with a counsellor. Although Maeve claimed that she was 'the happiest girl in the world' she gradually admitted that she was anxious about the wedding – booked for early June. Would her parents get on with Jason's? Suppose her pestilential little brother played up as usual? And the weather – if it rained . . .

Maeve could never admit that the discussions with the counsellor had made much difference but she had to agree that the dyspepsia was no longer the worry it had been.

Many sufferers find, like Maeve, that the standard indigestion medicines are ineffective but a brief course of mild sleeping tablets, such as temazepam, at least make the nights more bearable for those who have been waking in the small hours. If the symptoms of dyspepsia are bound up with anxiety or depression a combination of the talking treatment and the appropriate tablets will help.

Half the victims of biliary dyspepsia are cured by the removal of their gallbladder and another quarter are improved. However, this is a major operation, so it makes sense to find out what the chances are that you will be one of the lucky ones (see p. 45). Sometimes biliary dyspepsia develops when the gallbladder has already been removed, when it can be part of the post-cholecystectomy syndrome (see p. 32).

Because of the diversity of symptoms and causes which come under the umbrella of biliary dyspepsia, the treatment must sometimes address the individual symptoms as well as any underlying general problem.

Flatulence

Flatulence – hence *flatulent dyspepsia* – is a frequent complaint. Some 20 to 30 per cent of us suffer from dyspepsia at times and nearly always 'wind' is part of the syndrome, but it can stand as a disorder on its own. The essence is that you are uncomfortably aware of gas in your abdomen causing distension and tightness – bloating. After a meal, or even partway through, your belt needs loosening.

Eructation, burps and belching

These are due to gas escaping through your mouth, mainly from the oesophagus, not as we usually think, from the stomach. In some cultures a hostess is disappointed if her guests do not belch appreciatively at the table.

Air that is belched has been swallowed or more accurately, sucked in. Fizzy drinks enhance the tendency and some lager drinkers, especially, slurp in large volumes of liquid and air together. Talking non-stop while eating and drinking, or chewing gum – but not sucking sweets – have the same effect. Tense, anxious people can develop a habit of burping, perhaps to relieve a feeling of discomfort in their chest or abdomen, but the unnecessary burping can cause air to be swallowed, more discomfort and the genuine need to belch for relief. Ill-fitting dentures can make matters worse, but smoking makes no difference.

Some of the swallowed air passes down through the digestive system and escapes via the back passage, but most gas discharged that way originates in the intestines. A certain amount is normal. Two thousand years ago, among the Hippocratic axioms was one which stated that passing wind was necessary for well-being, while the Roman Emperor Claudius decreed that citizens should be allowed to pass air 'whenever necessary'. Nowadays we are embarrassed by what was taken for granted even a hundred years ago.

As with dyspepsia, if you are 45 or over when you start suffering from the burps and the farts, it is good sense to undergo a thorough MOT – to check for, for instance, peptic ulcer or pancreatitis. It is a help to understand where the gas comes from, and there are two medicines which help some people: either metoclopramide or cisapride, three times a day. The antacid preparations containing dimethicone are usually disappointing, although theoretically they should absorb the gas. Extra care not to bolt your meals half-chewed, or to chatter while putting in another forkful can make a surprising difference.

Occasionally troublesome burping is cured when a gastric ulcer, hiatus hernia – or gallstones – are diagnosed and treated effectively.

Bloating and excessive farting

These two symptoms go together and are often accompanied by embarrassingly loud borborygmi – tummy gurgles. Gas may collect in the caecum, where the small intestine joins the colon (see Figure 1). It makes a soft, squelchy, slightly tender swelling in the appendix area. Gas may also become trapped in the corner of the colon high up on the left of the abdomen under the spleen, giving pain in that part, or it may be distributed through the whole colon with more general discomfort.

The amount of flatus or wind that is passed below can vary between 200 and 2000 mls, but is normally around 600 ml, just under a pint. It consists of the gases carbon dioxide, methane and hydrogen which are all produced by the action of bacteria on food stuffs in the intestines. The main process is the fermentation of carbohydrates. These include lactose (milk sugar), lactulose (used as a laxative), wheat, corn, oats, potatoes and various other vegetables which we humans cannot properly digest. Obviously a diet containing a lot of these foods will encourage gas production.

Other foods liable to lead to flatulence include beans, nuts, raisins, onions, cabbage, Brussels sprouts, prunes and apples. Fructose and sorbitol act similarly; they are natural constituents in fruits, berries and many plants, and fructose (fruit sugar) is used as a sweetener in soft drinks.

Malabsorption is another cause of excessive fermentation in the gut, with abdominal discomfort and flatus and often diarrhoea. The inability to break down lactose is one common source of trouble, also the starches in wheat, rice, potatoes, bananas and beans. Coeliac disease and pancreatic disorders may be involved. People who go on the high fibre diets that are currently all the rage, and are specifically recommended for constipation and the irritable bowel syndrome, may incidentally increase their gas output. Floating motions are a sign that methane gas has been trapped in them.

Studies have shown that some people – most often young to middle-aged women – who may complain bitterly of distension and extreme discomfort in wearing clothes with a waistband or belt, show no objective evidence of excess gas in their intestines. They are bothered more by the bloating than by wind, especially before a period and in the evening. It seems that in women in particular the muscles of the colon may go slack as they do in pregnancy, but in these cases inappropriately. The relaxed colon can take up twice as much space as usual, making the abdomen bulge. This may be a reflex reaction to irritation somewhere else in the digestive system – even gallstones could be implicated. Those who feel the greatest discomfort, although they may have only slight swelling, have intestines which are extra-sensitive even to mild distension.

The tests to exclude serious trouble are the same as for belching with the addition of a cholecystogram. In general a low fibre diet is indicated, with avoidance of those of the foods listed which you discover, by trial and error, cause discomfort to you. Unless you really need them, antibiotics are best avoided.

The standard medicines are disappointing. Activated charcoal may be good for dogs with wind, but not for us, and dimethicone and kaolin are no better. Your main hope is to chew everything 32 times, like Gladstone, and experiment with your diet. It may also be worth trying the herbal remedy asafoetida, from the ancient Indian Ayurvedic culture. It smells like garlic, so the capsules are pleasanter to take than the liquid. The traditional Chinese treatment for bloating is magnolia bark – *hou po* – and orange peel. They come in tablet form.

Irritable bowel syndrome (IBS)

This is one of the commonest disorders of the digestive system in the West, affecting one in five women and one in 20 men in Britain. In the United States three times as many women as men are troubled by it and five times as many whites as blacks. This says something about the Western diet and lifestyle. In the Indian subcontinent, oddly enough, men with IBS outnumber the women.

The chief symptom is pain, for which your doctor can find no physical cause. Yet the syndrome consistently presents a characteristic set of symptoms, which are characteristically intermittent. Because they come and go, sufferers are always hopeful that this time the disorder has gone away for good and only about half of them consult their doctors. Probably the majority of ordinary, healthy women have some of the symptoms of IBS occasionally. Patients who attend gastroenterological clinics because of IBS tend to be more anxious and depressed than normal. This is not surprising when they are having bothersome symptoms and does not mean that they have neurotic personalities.

The symptoms include many of those seen in biliary dyspepsia and flatulence:

- Pain, ranging from 'severe', 'stabbing' or 'agonizing' to grumbling discomfort. It is usually at the front of the abdomen, any part, but it may seem to come from the back or the edge of the ribs. It is sometimes triggered by eating, especially a large, rich meal but often, fortunately, the pain only lasts a few minutes.
- Your usual bowel pattern is disrupted, sometimes towards constipation, but more often the motions become looser or variable.
- Passing a motion is sometimes urgent, and a humiliating accident can happen, but it is always a physical relief.
- You may feel that the bowel has not been completely emptied, but straining does not help – there is nothing there except possibly a few streaks of mucus.
- Distension of the abdomen after meal.
- Gurgling guts and excessive wind.
- Heartburn.
- Dyspepsia – biliary dyspepsia frequently includes the symptoms of IBS, and to a lesser extent vice versa.

Background: adults with irritable colon have often been plagued by 'tummy aches' as children, 'Little belly-achers grow up into big belly-achers.' Divorce, conflict, family disruption and even child abuse are more likely in the families of these children. IBS may truly be a 'gut reaction' to traumatic events. Current physical or psychological stress can also set off IBS. A change of diet, for instance on a foreign holiday is one such stress, or a slimming diet, which, interestingly, can also trigger true biliary colic. Other events occurring in the nine months before the onset of IBS often include the breakdown of a relationship, frequent family rows, or major ongoing problems at work.

Headaches or backache often accompany IBS and it is thought that this is due to powerful but poorly localized messages from the abdominal organs lighting up other branches of the nervous system.

Diets which contain too little bulk cause constipation. This may start IBS off, the constipated type. A low-fibre diet, consisting of cholesterol-rich junk food may increase the risk of IBS, but most sufferers eat normally and some are already taking the high-fibre option. Nevertheless food does have an influence.

Food intolerance is a controversial matter and testing for it is time-consuming, and to do it properly means going on to a strict elimination diet. This will stop the symptoms after a fortnight if some food is the trigger. Then, one by one, foods are reintroduced and if you hit the villain of your diet the symptoms return full-strength. You then know what to avoid. A full elimination test takes several months but there is a shortcut in IBS. Up to 70 per cent of sufferers find their symptoms improve if they omit all cereals except rice; also nuts, raisins, citrus fruits, onions, tea, coffee, alcohol, dairy products and all those convenience foods which contain additives – in fact many of the dishes we enjoy. It is then easy and quicker to try, cautiously, which foods you can take without ill effect. Food intolerance may not be the cause, but it occurs frequently in IBS.

A sigmoidoscopy is the most effective method of checking out your colon. The sigmoidoscope is a rigid, or more often today, a flexible fibreoptic instrument for looking into the bowel. It is useful, especially in an older person, to make sure there is no colon cancer. In irritable colon the only likely finding is an excess of mucus, and there is no increased risk of cancer.

There are four kinds of treatment for IBS, some of which apply to biliary dyspepsia without colonic symptoms.

1 Explanation and reassurance, since anxiety makes the symptoms worse.
2 Avoiding trouble-makers in your diet and equally in your social and work life: based on experience.
3 Stress management, counselling, aromatherapy, yoga, hypnosis – whatever best helps you to relax.

4 High fibre diet, possibly also a bulk laxative like Fybogel. Loose motions may need an anti-diarrhoeal such as Lomotil, or an antispasmodic like Colofac.

The most effective treatment of all for IBS is intensive psychotherapy.

6

Biliary dyskinesia

The whole digestive tract consists essentially of a tube with muscle fibres in its walls which tighten and relax rhythmically and in sequence to maintain a constant flow from the entrance – your mouth – to the exit – the anus. The arrival of meals, big or snack-size, from time to time causes variations in the speed of transit to allow for digestion. This means some precise timing in the muscle contractions.

A little further on than the stomach, in the duodenum, is a side branch from the biliary system which includes the gallbladder and the bile ducts. The gallbladder has a substantial amount of muscle in its wall and this contracts most vigorously after a meal, especially if it contained plenty of fat. A chemical messenger in the blood – the hormone, cholecystokinin, is produced in response to the presence of food and in turn acts as a trigger to the gallbladder's pushing out its store of bile. The gallbladder's contractions operate in conjunction with the opening of the sphincter of Oddi, a muscular ring guarding the exit of the common bile duct into the duodenum. The purpose is to release bile into the duodenum when there is food waiting there requiring digestion, particularly of fats.

Functional disorders of the digestive tract are those in which there are symptoms but no abnormalities in the digestive organs themselves: oesophagus, stomach, biliary system, duodenum and the rest of the intestines, small and large. Some of the causes relating to dyspepsia have been outlined in Chapter 5. Another major cause is a fault in the timing of the muscular activity so that particular sections, including the muscle of a sphincter, tighten up and go into spasm inappropriately instead of smoothly, harmoniously and in synchrony. This faulty, jerky muscular movement is called *dyskinesia* (*dys-* bad, *-kinesia* movement). So-called biliary dyskinesia may be due to faulty contraction or lack of contraction affecting the gallbladder itself, or mistiming of the opening or closing of one of two sphincters. They are the pyloric sphincter, where the oesophagus joins the stomach, and the sphincter of Oddi, gate-keeper to the duodenum. If the pyloric sphincter relaxes inappropriately, when the stomach is full, heartburn results from the stomach acid irritating the delicate lining of the oesophagus.

Wherever there is muscle spasm, there is pain in the muscle itself, apart from its holding back material that should be moving down the alimentary tract. This may include small stones. Tension builds in the dammed-up fluid, for instance bile in the gallbladder or bile ducts. Unfortunately the pain or discomfort you feel and are able to relay to your doctor is a poor guide for distinguishing gallbladder pain from other causes of abdominal pain.

The Cholecystokinin Provocation Test helps. This consists in observing the results of an injection of cholecystokinin. If the gallbladder is the seat of pain due to faulty contractions, the injection will bring on the exact pain the person has been experiencing – a positive result. This indicates gallbladder dyskinesia, and gives the go-ahead for cholecystectomy – surgical removal of the gallbladder. There is then a good chance that the pain will be gone for good. When there is dyspepsia with a negative cholecystokinin test, the operation is contraindicated. It would involve the trauma and risks of major surgery with little prospect of a successful outcome.

Dawn

Dawn, aged 45, was a strong character. She had been 'a martyr to her stomach' by which she meant her abdomen in general, for four or five years. She had frequent nausea and almost continuous pain in the upper abdomen which became sharply worse if she ate a fatty meal. Her doctor felt that the fatty meal was almost as good a test as cholecystokinin and referred her to the hospital with a recommendation for a cholecystectomy.

The surgeon refused. In the course of the preliminary investigations it emerged that Dawn was sensitive to lactose – milk sugar. A diet free from all dairy produce, including, of course, cheese and butter, led to a gradual improvement in her symptoms.

While overactivity – *hyperkinesia* – of the gallbladder muscles can cause pain, so may poor, weak contractions – *hypokinesia*. This allows the gallbladder to fill up with mucus and bile, producing irritation of the mucous membrane lining and tension in the whole organ. The cholecystokinin test will be negative in such cases, but ultrasound examination will show changes in the size of the gallbladder as it empties appropriately or not, and a radionuclide test assesses the amount of bile it passes out. It may be that a very narrow cystic duct is impeding the flow from the gallbladder and causing tension. Removal of the gallbladder would put an end to the symptoms.

The sphincter of Oddi

This is the muscle ring guarding the doorway from the common bile duct into the duodenum. It is also subject to dyskinesia.

Thelma

Thelma was 50 when she had her gallbladder removed. It was full of stones, but the surgeon was confident that none had been left behind. After four or five pain-free years Thelma began having recurrent attacks of pain like biliary colic. It was just like the pain she had before the operation – but now she had no gallbladder. There was no evidence of stones now, and blood tests (amylase and liver enzymes) put her pancreas and liver in the clear.

That left the sphincter of Oddi in the frame. To check whether it was contracting and relaxing as it should, an ultrasound investigation was made to see if there was any hold-up in the biliary system after Thelma had eaten a fried meal. The common bile duct looked wider than normal which suggested this might be the case, but a better test was the endoscopic one. The endoscope (a fibreoptic tube with a manometer attachment) was passed through Thelma's mouth down the digestive tract where it was used to measure the pressure of the bile at the sphincter of Oddi. Thelma was sedated.

The reading was just over 40mg of mercury, indicating stenosis of the sphincter – scar tissue surrounded it so that it could not relax properly. It was the back pressure in the bile duct which was at the root of Thelma's pain. The answer was a sphincterotomy – cutting the fibrous tissue to open up the sphincter and release the pressure. This minor procedure was carried out simply and quickly via the endoscope, although an open operation was an option if there had been any difficulty. Thelma's pain was relieved almost at once and did not return. The scarring had probably arisen when the area was inflammed by cholecystitis or possibly damaged by a stone which had since passed on.

Stenosis means a narrowing and stiffening with fibrous tissue so that the muscle can neither tighten nor loosen. Other reasons for an inefficient sphincter include spontaneous bursts of rapid contractions, producing short-lived obstruction to the flow of bile. This is due to an irritable sphincter which may also lead to longer-lasting muscular spasms. The manometric (pressure) readings reveal the situation. Occasionally the sphincter of Oddi reacts paradoxically to the normal, after-meal release of cholecystokinin and contracts instead of relaxing. The flow of bile is dammed up and the back pressure causes pain. This abnormal response to cholecystokinin can be demonstrated by the test.

None of the numerous medicines which have been tried consistently relieves the pain from an intermittently blocked sphincter and sphincterotomy which is so successful for stenosis is only helpful in a few of these cases.

Irritable bowel, which can mimic biliary dyspepsia or be part of the syndrome, is also thought to be in part, at least, due to dyskinesia. Sections of colon may clench intermittently, like a fist, resulting in the characteristic symptoms either of blockage of the colon – constipation, or accelerated transit of its contents – diarrhoea.

Since mental tension induces and enhances muscle tension, especially in the internal organs, if you are suffering from symptoms that could be due to dyskinesia, it is worth while reviewing your lifestyle for stress points and ironing out any ongoing areas of conflict.

Part II
Some answers

7

Checking out: investigations

Gallstones usually do no harm so long as they stay within the gallbladder and do not get too large or too crowded. The trouble starts when they sneak out and cause you pain and maybe damage by landing up in the wrong place. Your doctor, of course, cannot give you effective treatment unless he or she finds out exactly what has gone wrong, where and why. The areas under suspicion include the gallbladder itself, the cystic, common bile and hepatic ducts and, secondarily, the pancreas and liver.

The big snag is that almost all problems involving gallstones or the gallbladder produce the same basic symptom complex: biliary colic. The presence of jaundice sheds a little extra light, but the major obstacle is that you cannot see what is going on inside the abdomen – at least not with the naked eye. Back in the nineteenth century there was nothing to help the doctor's naked eye. Drs Wickham Legg and Thudicum, around 1890, had only one piece of technology – a sieve. The idea was to check for gallstones by sieving the motions, where, apart from sizable specimens, gravel would indicate the presence of stones. No wonder they felt chary about advising their patients. 'The physician can never speak confidently when treating a case he *looks upon as one of gallstones*.'

Nowadays, and especially in the last decade, although there is no direct test for gallstones, we have a range of methods for revealing the secrets previously hidden in the abdomen. We cannot quite open a door and look inside, but we have next best in our modern imaging techniques: sophisticated X-rays, ultrasound, and computerized tomography, backed up by biochemical tests. Nevertheless, the first and most important source of information for the doctor is YOU – what you feel and how your body is functioning. Chapter 4 covers this aspect.

The tests

Blood tests

These may be a useful preliminary, for instance in checking for cholestatis. The sluggish flow of bile, a major contributor to stone

51

formation, may be due to impaired production because of a liver disorder, or to obstruction in a bile duct, usually by a stone.

Liver function tests

These indicate whether the problem is in the liver cells or the biliary network:

- high, fluctuating levels of bilirubin in the plasma indicate blockage by a stone; it will also show in jaundice and dark urine;
- high aminotransferase levels indicate liver cells in trouble, for instance with inflammation which may have been started by gallstones;
- high alkaline phosphatase levels mean obstruction;
- transaminases are enzymes released into the blood when liver cells have been damaged. They reflect inflammation in the liver, including cholangitis set off by a gallstone (see p. 24).

Leucocytosis

Leucocytosis, a large number of white cells in the blood, is a defence mechanism associated with infection of the liver or the gallbladder.

Urine test for bilirubin

This is a simple dipstick test. A sliver of wood or card, suitably impregnated, is dipped into a specimen of urine and changes colour if bilirubin is present, which occurs in obstructive jaundice (see p. 23).

Plain X-ray

What this can reveal:

- The 10–30 per cent of gallstones that show up because of their calcium content. They are called radio-opaque. Almost all black pigment stones are radio-opaque, but almost none of the brown; cholesterol stones may be. Stones which do not show on X-ray are radiolucent.
- Deposits of calcium in the wall of the gallbladder – porcelain gallbladder (see p. 30).
- Calcium in the pancreas area indicates chronic pancreatitis (see p. 24).
- Gas, which looks dark, in the bile system may be because of emphysematous cholecystitis (see p. 28) or a false passage between the gallbladder and the intestine, where a stone has eroded through.

- An inflamed gallbladder – cholecystitis – appears as a soft mass.
- Cyst, abscess or tumour of the liver may make a shadow on the film.

Oral cholecystography

This is a method of making the gallbladder and bile ducts show up in an X-ray. The trick is to take, by mouth a contrast agent, a chemical which is taken up by the liver and then concentrated, with the bile, in the gallbladder. The gallbladder and its ducts then stand out white on the film, revealing their layout and any abnormalities. Radiolucent stones appear as dark spaces in the bile, but it can be difficult to spot radio-opaque stones against it. The tablets used in cholecystography are all iodine compounds: Telepaque, Biloptin and Solubiloptin. They are all equally effective.

Mary

Mary was 53. In the last six weeks she had experienced two attacks of acute abdominal pain and nausea after a rich meal, and her doctor wanted to check the possibility of gallstones. He arranged for her to have an oral cholecystogram (oral – by mouth, cholecyst – gallbladder, gram – picture or diagram). This was the form:

1 A day or two before the test Mary had a plain abdominal X-ray, to pick up any radio-opaque stones before she had taken any of the contrast agent which could 'hide' them.
2 The night before the test she was asked to have a plain, non-fatty supper and then to fast overnight.
3 On the next day, over a period of 12 hours, Mary took measured amounts of Biloptin, her doctor's choice of contrast agent, because it has the best record for few side-effects. The total dose, calculated on her weight, was approximately 5 gram.
4 During the 12 hours Mary had to drink at least 2 litres of fluid, but avoiding milk because of its fat content.
5 Mary was X-rayed several times in the day, standing up and lying on her front and her back at different angles to make sure of a good view of every part of the vital area. Multiple tiny stones would be easiest to detect in the films where she was standing upright – they would float on top of the bile, making a horizontal line across the gallbladder.
6 Finally, Mary had a fatty meal (she chose fish and chips and a

chocolate gateau) to stimulate her gallbladder to contract. This propelled enough of the radio-opaque bile into the common bile duct to give a good picture of that, too. It may not show well otherwise.

Mary's cholecystogram revealed several stones in the gallbladder and one in the cystic duct, the probable culprit causing her pain.

Interpreting the results: after the contrast agent gets to the liver, the concentrated bile in the gallbladder makes it show up white in the X-ray. If this does not happen the test process is repeated next day. If the gallbladder still remains invisible it indicates that it is not functioning. This may be because of a stone in Hartmann's pouch at the neck of the gallbladder or in the cystic duct blocking it off. If there is a marked excess of bilirubin in the bile from the liver cells, the patient will be jaundiced and the test will not work.

An oral cholecystogram picks up 92–95 per cent of gallstones, and is generally safe. Mary was lucky, but a third of those undergoing the test have minor but unwelcome side-effects from the contrast agent: nausea, vomiting, diarrhoea or a rash. Serious side effects are exceptional. A bonus is information on the motility of the gallbladder, as demonstrated after the fatty meal.

Ultrasound examination

This imaging technique is simple, quick and comfortable and so safe that it is used routinely in pregnancy. For the last dozen years it has been the front runner in the investigation of disorders related to gallstones, with a detection rate for stones of 98 per cent.

The principle: a hand-held probe which emits ultrasound waves, which we cannot hear, is held against the skin over the liver and gallbladder area. These waves bounce off various objects in their line of fire. Bats as well as aircraft use this method for navigation.

The ultrasound waves are converted by a transducer into a visible film – with stills. Solid objects, such as stones or the junction between two surfaces, come out white and are said to give a 'bright' echo. There are dark sound shadows behind them, if they are solid.

The procedure

The best time to do an ultrasound examination is first thing in the morning, after fasting all night. At this time there is the least chance of gas in the intestines blurring the picture, while on the other hand the gallbladder is normally full and readily visualized by the apparatus. The test itself consists of a large number of transverse and longitudinal scans made over the gallbladder area, sliding the probe across the skin, which has previously been anointed with oil. The transverse scans in particular are needed to detect the smallest stones.

What ultrasound scanning of the biliary system can show

- Gallstones, whatever their composition, down to a minimum size of 2 mm in diameter. Stones must be seen to shift their position during a film, unlike cysts, polyps or other tumours which are anchored to the gallbladder.
- The gallbladder, including the thickness of its walls – increased by scar tissue and enlarged muscles in chronic cholecystitis.
- Cancer of the pancreas, a cause of misdiagnosis; also chronic pancreatitis.
- Ballooning of a bile duct, indicating an obstruction (usually by a stone) and its position. The maximum diameter for a healthy bile duct is 6 mm, but there is a general increase in width with age or after removal of the gallbladder.
- Sludge shows up as a bright echo, but does not cast a sound shadow – bleeding into the gallbladder appears similar.
- Gas from gas-forming bacteria or a fistula shows black.
- Abscesses, cysts or tumours of the liver show on ultrasound, if they are 5 cm across or more.

If the gallbladder cannot be seen in an ultrasound film it may be because it has become a small shrunken scrap of scar tissue from chronic inflammation, or it is so full of stones that there is no room for the bile to make a contrast. In these cases the old-fashioned oral cholecystogram comes into its own or the more modern, computerized tomography.

George

'Your tan is fading already,' said his wife. George had just returned from a golfing trip to the Algarve with six other enthusiasts from his firm. He felt disappointingly under par – and not in the golfing sense. Before the holiday he had been frightened by a sharp attack of pain like a band round his chest. He – and his doctor – thought he was having a heart attack, but an electrocardiogram showed his heart to be working normally, and anyway the pain had passed.

While they were away, getting loads of fresh air and exercise, 'the chaps' had huge appetites. George, like the others, ate and drank more than usual and 'had to pay for it' with bloating, nausea and often a sharp pain. It was not until his wife's remark that he realized that not only his face, but the whites of his eyes were a dingy, brownish yellow.

Ultrasound showed ballooning of the common bile duct – an indication of obstruction by a stone. The label attached to George's condition was *choledocholithiasis*: *chole* – bile, *docho* – duct, *lithiasis* – stone formation. He had the operation on his 59th birthday – endoscopic sphincterotomy.

Computerized tomography

CT scanning provides a series of X-ray pictures which look as though the body had been cut in slices 1 centimetre apart. It is more expensive and takes more time than ultrasound, but is useful when the latter gives an equivocal result. Any part of the body can be scanned in fair detail by CT, but it is not as good as ultrasound in detecting the smallest stones. Some 76 per cent of bile duct stones are caught by CT, if the duct is dilated, but in the 20 per cent of cases where the duct is of normal width it does not give a reliable result.

CT is particularly helpful in some fistulae (false passages) because it shows the presence of gas (see p. 52).

Radionuclide scanning (cholescintigraphy)

This investigation employs a chemical with a temporary radioactive tag which is taken up rapidly and exclusively by the liver, and then passed on into the bile duct system.

Irene

Pain, nausea and jaundice and a cold sweat had gripped Irene without warning. When the pain and nausea had subsided her doctor arranged for her to have a radionuclide scan, because this method is still effective in the presence of jaundice. Irene had to fast for four hours minimum – four and a quarter, to be sure, then a solution of radio-tagged iminodiacetic acid was injected into a vein in her arm. The relevant area was scanned with a gamma camera, to pick up the radiation.

Results

The bile ducts usually become visible in 10–15 minutes. The gallbladder and duodenum begin to show in about half-an-hour. If the gallbladder is not visualized within an hour the test is said to be positive. This means that the gallbladder is blocked off from the rest of the system – invariably the case in acute cholecystitis. Radionuclide testing is the best for investigating the cystic duct, and identifies 98–100 per cent of cases of acute cholecystitis. However, the test is also positive in 82 per cent of all those suffering from biliary colic. Ultrasound is quicker.

Endoscopic retrograde cholangiopancreatography (ERCP)

Endoscopy means looking inside the body, physically. In this investigation it is combined with an X-ray film of what is seen.

Procedure

1 An explanation of what is going to happen and why.
2 You are sedated with injections into a vein (intravenous) of pethidine and midazolam, a relative of Valium, also an injection of atropine to dry up your saliva.
3 You lie on your left side with your left arm behind you.
4 An anaesthetic spray is applied to the back of your throat, the only part involved which is sensitive.
5 The duodenoscope is slipped down your gullet. In this fibreoptic instrument, flexible fibres carry light waves.
6 A dose of hyoscine relaxes the duodenum, and the sphincter of Oddi is relaxed by a spray under the tongue of glycerol trinitrate (see Figure 1.1).
7 Contrast medium is slowly injected through the sphincter directly into the common bile duct (it can also be injected into the pancreatic duct if the pancreas is to be examined).
8 Serial X-rays are taken and developed immediately: the whole of the biliary tree of ducts and the gallbladder are outlined. The bile duct appears larger by this method than with ultrasound.
9 For the last few X-rays of the gallbladder you lie on your back.

Results

There is a 98 per cent success rate in detecting gallstones in the bile ducts with this method as well as information about the gallbladder. Complications are uncommon, less than 1 in 100, and usually

57

amount to a brief, mild attack of pancreatitis. However, it takes a high degree of skill to carry out the investigation, and sometimes it fails.

Percutaneous transhepatic cholangiography (PTA)

This method of examination is used if ERCP is unsuccessful. The name incorporates 'through the skin' – percutaneous, 'across the liver' – transhepatic and 'picturing the bile duct' cholangiography. In essence, a fine needle is passed through the liver into the common bile duct under a local anaesthetic and a radio-opaque chemical is injected. The whole process is continuously monitored by X-ray. The needle, named a 'skinny', is just over half a millimetre in diameter, comprising a removable stylus inside a hollow canal for the injection fluid.

As prophylaxis, since infection is the main risk, you are given an intravenous injection of antibiotic, probably a cephalosporin, before the procedure is started. An injection, also into a vein, of the minor tranquillizer, midazolam, makes you comfortably drowsy throughout.

Results

There is a 98 per cent success rate in visualizing the bile ducts, gallbladder and any stones, if the bile duct is dilated (for this method the maximum normal width is 7.5 mm). With a bile duct of normal width the detection rate falls to 70 per cent.

This method is particularly effective in *recurrent pyogenic cholangitis* when the stones are in the bile ducts within the liver. These are likely to be the brown pigment stones most commonly found in the Far East.

Intravenous cholangiography

As with radionuclide scanning this method involves an intravenous injection of a substance which shows up, in this case on a type of X-ray.

Procedure

As shown for Leslie, who had suffered from recurrent biliary colic for two years, although his gallbladder had been removed by keyhole surgery. Neither ERCP nor PTA had worked out satisfactorily.

Leslie

As soon as the idea of the intravenous method was mooted, Leslie's consultant asked him if he had any liver or kidney problems, asthma or heart disease or was sensitive to iodine. He did not need to ask him about pregnancy. Any of these would have been contraindications to the examination and some other method would have been sought. The test does not work if the patient has jaundice, but Leslie did not.

Before the test began the decks were cleared by fasting at one end and an enema to clear the colon at the other. Then an infusion of an iodine compound, the contrast agent, was slowly run into a vein at Leslie's elbow, taking half to three-quarters of an hour for 100 mls. Tomographs – slice-like vertical X-rays were taken after the infusion and again 1–3 hours later to show the gallbladder and finally 24 hours later to detect the layering of stones of different sizes and types in the gallbladder.

In Leslie's case a stone was found in the common bile duct and removed surgically.

Results

In those without any sign of jaundice and a normal level of bilirubin in their serum this method gives a reasonably good picture of the bile ducts in up to 90 per cent of patients, but falls to 10 per cent with higher levels. The detection rate for stones is not as good as with direct cholangiography, and it fails to show up as many as 50 per cent of stones revealed by an oral cholecystogram.

It is mainly used after a cholecystectomy and when ERCP and PTA have failed, but some hospitals use it routinely to check for stones before the operation.

Liver biopsy

This method of checking up on the liver means passing a needle into the liver below the lower ribs on the right side of the body, and sucking out a small sample of tissue. A local anaesthetic is put in by injection, but it can be uncomfortable having a relatively large needle inserted. Liver biopsy helps in assessing the degree of inflammation or any other liver disorder, but it is seldom needed in the diagnosis of gallstone problems.

These are just some of the ways of finding out whether or not you have gallstones and if they are up to any mischief, but there are constant updates and improvements. One such is EUS – endoscopic ultrasound, in which the ultrasound probe functions from inside the body, and there are plenty more.

8

Treatment 1: non-surgical

There have been fantastic advances in medical technology in the last quarter century. These have revolutionized the range and sophistication of the treatments available for dealing with disorders due to gallstones. Among the most remarkable are the telescopes for viewing internal organs, in which light travels along twisting, flexible fibres – seeing round corners is standard. Then there are the tiny camcorders to slip inside the abdomen through an incision a few millimetres long which throw their picture on to a full-size television screen for the surgeon to chart the operation. And the chemists unravelling biological secrets to make designer drugs.

The choice is wide and diverse, but the trick is to match the particular treatment to individual circumstances.

The do-nothing ploy

This is one choice in the case of 'silent' gallstones, which have usually been discovered by chance in an X-ray for some unrelated problem, or in the course of an abdominal operation, for instance for appendicitis or peptic ulcer. The point about these stones is that they have not advertised their presence, and even when you and your doctor know about them, they are giving you no grief. On the principle 'If it's not broke, don't mend it,' most gastroenterologists opt for doing nothing. Only a minority of silent gallstones will ever cause problems and even then, nothing urgent or dangerous is likely.

Everyone agrees that symptoms call for treatment, and there are special circumstances when the 'do nothing' rule needs to be overridden. In Pima Indians and Chileans the presence of gallstones carries a much greater risk of gallbladder cancer than in other ethnic groups, more so as they get older. Similarly, larger gallstones increase the cancer risk in all races. With stones of more than 3 mm across it rises by 10 per cent. In these cases it makes good sense to remove the gallbladder, especially since this is a very safe operation nowadays, and with keyhole surgery means only a few days in hospital.

Now that there are such neat manoeuvres for removing the

gallstones without the gallbladder, some specialists believe they should rid their patients of any gallstones discovered, however harmless they seem. The expense of providing treatment unless it is strictly necessary weighs with health service managers, but doctors and patients may feel differently.

General measures

When biliary colic does not resolve spontaneously within an hour or so, the first line of treatment is bed rest, a warm pad or hot water bottle to the painful area, and pain relief. If paracetamol does not touch it an injection into the muscle of pethidine (100 mg) or pentazocine (30 mg) may be needed every two to three hours. An atropine injection also helps by relaxing the sphincter of Oddi, reducing any back pressure on the gallbladder, and most people need an anti-emetic injection, which has the added benefit of being mentally calming, too. It is very likely that you will be transferred to hospital, if the symptoms have not passed off in an hour or two.

If the pain is still not reasonably well under control the analgesia is upgraded to morphine – it is clear by this stage that acute inflammation has set in, and possibly infection. Morphine can make you feel nauseated, despite the anti-sickness medicine, and for anyone who cannot stop vomiting a nasogastric tube brings relief. A thin, flexible tube is slipped into one nostril down into the stomach and its contents aspirated. This is not as uncomfortable as it sounds – I know, I have had it.

Because it is important that you do not become dehydrated while you may not be able to keep any drink down, a saline drip is put into a vein at your elbow, and any unpleasant sensation of thirst is abolished. Antibiotics are also given intravenously if you are a senior citizen, have jaundice or a high temperature. The cephalosporins are useful catch-all bug-killers, and one of these is usually backed up by another antibiotic, metronidazole (Flagyl) given in a suppository.

When it has become clear that cholecystitis has developed you will be advised that you must part with your gallbladder, sooner or later. *Sooner* means within hours or a couple of days of the attack. *Later* refers to a delay of 10 to 15 days (for the surgical details, see p. 70). It is unwise and unsafe, even if this attack subsides completely, to rely on medical treatment indefinitely once you have had an inflamed gallbladder. Further attacks are a certainty and will probably be more severe.

Medical treatments which remove the stones but leave the gallbladder

The obvious snag is that the stones may recur. This is less likely if the original cause was temporary, for example pregnancy, taking oestrogen medication, clofibrate, spironolactone, phenobarbitone or a major tranquillizer, or going through a period of excessively strict slimming.

Oral dissolution

This involves taking medicine by mouth which will dissolve the stones while they are in the gallbladder. Unfortunately this attractive-sounding method is only suitable for 30 per cent of stones – small cholesterol ones only, which contain little or no calcium, and are radiolucent, that is they do not show up in an X-ray. The maximum manageable size is 15 mm in diameter. The gallbladder must be in good working order, filling and emptying appropriately and free from inflammation or any acute symptoms. This involves checking by oral cholecystography (see p. 53). Personal factors, such as obesity or unwillingness to stick to the course for the mandatory year or more, cut the number of patients completing the course by two-thirds.

The medication, consisting of capsules or tablets of bile acids, is taken once in the 24 hours, most conveniently at night.

There are three regimes:

1 *Chenodeoxycholic acid*: this occurs naturally and in 1972 was observed by Dr Danziger and his colleagues to have the power of dissolving stones. It works in two ways, by suppressing the synthesis of cholesterol in the liver, the raw material of stones, and also decreasing the amount absorbed in the small intestine. Chenodeoxycholic acid has potentially toxic side-effects, but fortunately it is almost all eliminated in the motions. The one troublesome result is diarrhoea, which affects 30–60 per cent of those taking it, depending on the size of the dose. In all cases this is worked out on the weight of the patient. Only a small minority of sufferers are treated by chenodeoxycholic acid alone.

2 *Ursodeoxycholic acid (Urdox, Ursofalk, Destolit)*: this also occurs naturally, but is twice as expensive as chenodeoxycholic acid, since only half of the dose is absorbed. It does not have the potential for side-effects, and its mode of action is different – but less effective. It does not suppress the production of cholesterol, but it does impede its absorption, and it holds back the formation of cholesterol crystals, often the starting point of a stone. This is the usual choice if only one bile acid is given, but a popular approach is to take both.

3 *Combination treatment*: this is a mix of both bile acids in equal dosage – 5–7 mg of each, instead of a much higher dose of just one. The dose of chenodeoxycholic acid is now too small to cause side-effects and the combination method costs 25 per cent less than Urdox alone.

Even when the stones are the right size, not too numerous and all made of cholesterol, and the patient is not overweight or taking any incompatible medication, there are big disadvantages with oral dissolution therapy.

First, it takes so long – a year is the minimum treatment time. Second, for a woman it means avoiding pregnancy throughout this period, and using some other contraception than the Pill. For stones of 5–10 mm diameter, 1–2 years will be required to dissolve them, but smaller stones may need only 6–12 months. It will be longer if you put on weight and are more than 10 per cent above the average for your height and sex. Your body becomes resistant to the medication and you may need double the dose, with an added risk of side-effects. Third, there is the risk of recurrence during the next two or three years.

In a perfect patient, who plays it by the book for as long as it takes, there is a 60 per cent likelihood of success with the method, but a more realistic figure is probably 30–40 per cent for those on chenodeoxycholic acid and only 20–30 per cent for those taking ursodeoxycholic acid alone. The combination treatment can give you a flying start, but then progress slows down. No regime is quicker than any other in the end.

Throughout the treatment period you have six-monthly checks by ultrasound or oral cholecystography. It usually takes six months before the tests show any reduction in the size of the stones, but if there is no change at all after a year there is little point in continuing. It is not surprising that this long-drawn-out process had been almost abandoned, except for those with such serious health problems – usually heart or lung – that they cannot take the risk of anaesthesia and surgery. However, the introduction of *shock-wave lithotripsy*, which can break gallstones up into small pieces while they are still in the body, has given a new stimulus to the use of bile acid therapy (see p. 63). Everyone having lithotripsy takes a course of bile acids, starting before the procedure and continuing until all the fragments of stone have disappeared.

Rowachol treatment

Rowachol is a preparation in olive oil containing six related chemicals, *monoturpines*, of which the best known is menthol. It prevents the formation of cholesterol crystals and so impedes the development of gallstones. It can be given on its own or in combination with bile acids, for a similar length of time. This and some other drugs, Lovastatin and Simvastatin, are promising additions to the drug treatment of gallstones, but require further research into their safety and efficacy.

Direct contact dissolution

Gallbladder stones

In this method the dissolving chemical is poured directly on to the stones. A liquid relative of the anaesthetic gas, ether, is very effective in dissolving cholesterol stones, and their size or number is no bar to success. Unfortunately it does not work on calcium or pigment. The liquid is introduced into the gallbladder through a long needle, under X-ray monitoring. A sedative and a local anaesthetic make the process painless if not pleasurable.

Stones in the common bile duct

To deal with these a sticky mix of glycerol compounds is dribbled into the common bile duct through an endoscope, a flexible, self-lighting tube running from one nostril, through the sphincter of Oddi into the bile duct. At a slow drip of 3–5 ml per hour, the tube needs to remain in place for about three weeks – an unpleasant experience with a high risk of side-effects. Say 'no' if it is offered to you.

Extracorporeal shock-wave lithotripsy

This comprises shattering gallstones inside the body by focusing electrical shock waves on them from outside (*extra*) the body (*corporeal*). *Litho* just means stone. This form of treatment has been in use for decades for dealing with kidney stones, but its first successful application to gallstones was not until 1986. It has since proved to be a relatively safe and effective procedure, mostly used in conjunction with bile acids (see above). In its early days, the treatment used to be very uncomfortable, but nowadays it is completely painless. It only takes half-an-hour on an outpatient basis and then you can go home.

The procedure

You lie on a special table, face downwards for gallbladder stones, and on your back for a stone in the common bile duct. The location of the gallstones is shown by ultrasound so that the lithotriptor (wave generator) can be focused correctly. The best results depend on the accuracy of this focusing. The stones are reduced to gravel which is easily dissolved with bile acid therapy, usually started a week before the lithotripsy. This treatment is not suitable for everybody.

What you must have for this type of lithotripsy with gallbladder stones:

- symptoms of biliary colic, now or past;
- a normal, working gallbladder, demonstrated by oral cholecystography (see p. 53);
- one to three stones, with a total diameter of more than 30 mm;
- very little calcification, as seen in an X-ray.

What you should not have in the case of gallbladder stones:

- aspirin or an anticoagulant medicine such as warfarin;
- non-steroidal anti-inflammatory medication (NSAIDs), often used for pain relief in arthritis and rheumatism;
- allergy to X-ray contrast agents, for instance iodine used in the oral cholecystogram taken before and after the treatment;
- liver disease;
- pregnancy;
- pacemaker or serious heart disease;
- peptic ulcer;
- acute cholecystitis or other acute inflammation in the biliary system;
- acute pancreatitis;
- stones in the common bile duct.

It is a disadvantage to be overweight, for this as for so much in life.

There are several designs of lithotriptor. In general those which are least likely to cause side-effects may need the treatment to be repeated two or three times to be effective. A slight fever immediately after the shock is the commonest side-effect. It soon passes, as do the tiny flecks of haemorrhage (petechiae) which sometimes appear in the skin following the treatment.

Jessica

Jessica suffered considerable pain from one large gallstone that was stuck just before the place where the cystic duct joined the common bile duct. Her gallbladder was chronically inflamed from the partial blockage. Although an endoscope tube could be passed through the duodenum into the common bile duct it was considered too big to pass into the cystic duct, so the percutaneous route was chosen.

Local anaesthetic numbed Jessica's skin where the needle was inserted, and she had the heady feeling of floating in and out of a dream, the effect of midazolam, a calming medicine. The exact position of the stone was located by ultrasound and it was broken up by lithotripsy and the tiny pieces sucked out through the needle track. Jessica was amazed that her abdominal pain left her almost as soon as the stone was gone. Free from the intermittent and increasing back pressure, Jessica's gallbladder and ducts were no longer irritated and the inflammation subsided.

The ultimate non-surgical method of dealing with gallbladder stones is either so-called chemical cholecystectomy, which destroys the lining of the gallbladder so that it can no longer make stones, or diathermy ablation of the cystic duct, which has the same effect. These procedures are seldom necessary.

Treatment of bile duct stones

Extracorporeal shock-wave lithotripsy

This can be applied, with the patient lying face upwards. Other forms of lithotripsy, suitable for large stones, are ultrasonic, laser or a mechanical rotational type: these are used mainly for people who do not want or cannot safely have the general anaesthetic needed for the surgical removal of a stone. A solvent to clear up the gravelly fragments can be introduced through a nasobiliary tube, inserted during ERCP (endoscopic retrograde cholangiopancreatography). The percutaneous approach, passing a wide-bore needle through the skin (as happened with Jessica), has the advantage that bits of stone can be extracted mechanically via the needle track, ridding you of all traces of it straight away.

Intracorporeal lithotripsy

This process means introducing a lithotriptor into the abdomen through an endoscope, placed as near the stone or stones as possible. The surgeon can work by the endoscope light.

Endoscopic sphincterotomy

The most favoured methods today for removing stones in the common bile duct are the percutaneous route, as in Jessica's case, or cutting the muscular ring of the sphincter of Oddi and getting the stone out directly. This method is considered the best in particular circumstances:

- after the gallbladder has been removed;
- before keyhole surgery on the gallbladder;
- when the bile ducts from the liver are inflamed: cholangitis;
- when acute pancreatitis has been caused by a gallstone;
- with Mirizzi's syndrome (see p. 31).

Antibiotic therapy

Numerous bacteria are found normally in the digestive tract, but not in the gallbladder. In the case of obstruction casual neighbourhood bacteria may become trapped, causing an infection. Those most likely to be involved are:

- *Escherichia (E.) coli*;
- *Streptococci*;
- *Klebsiella*;
- *Pseudomonas*.

And less often:

- *Staphylococci*;
- *Haemophilus influenzae*.

And two which live without air and produce gas in the body:

- *Bacteroides*;
- *Clostridium*.

Whenever you have surgery affecting the biliary system you will have an antibiotic before, during and after the operation. With such a wide range of potential enemies, you will need a wide-spectrum antibiotic, that is one that deals with several strains. Those most often used are:

- Cephalosporins;
- Penicillins;
- Gentamycin;
- Metronidazole.

9

Treatment 2: surgical

More people than ever are suffering because of gallstones, and cholecystitis (inflammation of the gallbladder) is now the commonest reason for a major abdominal operation, outstripping both appendicitis and peptic ulcer.

Cholecystectomy

Surgical removal of the gallbladder is the only effective treatment for cholecystitis, acute or chronic. The operation comes in two styles – ancient and modern or incisional or laparoscopic.

Incisional cholecystectomy

This operation has a hundred years' hallowed history and is still the standard treatment. It involves making a cut in the abdomen large enough to expose the area containing the gallbladder and to allow the surgeon room to manipulate normal-sized instruments. This operation has become an extremely safe procedure, with fewer than 5 per cent of the patients having any trouble at all after the surgery, and a mortality of less than one in a thousand in those under 50, rising slightly with advancing age. When problems do arise they are usually due to heart and artery problems, chest disease or a sick liver rather than to the surgery.

Improvements brought in during the last 25 years include:

- advances in anaesthetics;
- better post-operative care;
- X-ray monitoring, which greatly reduces the risk of leaving stones in the common bile duct, a common cause of problems after the operation;
- techniques for removing errant stones spotted at the time of the cholecystectomy.

Mini-incisional cholecystectomy

This is practised by many surgeons today, an open operation but using a smaller incision than previously. The healing time is reduced and the scar smaller.

Laparoscopic cholecystectomy

This modern method – keyhole surgery – is now widely applied. It depends on the near magic of fibreoptics and the miniaturization of such complex instruments as television cameras and telescopes. The telescope or video camera is introduced into the abdomen by a tiny cut in the skin just below the navel. In the first case the surgeon will operate under direct vision through the telescope, and in the second from the image thrown onto a full-size TV screen by the tiny camcorder. The instruments are especially adapted and small, and reach the gallbladder through small nicks in the skin of the abdomen. Usually three or four of these are needed.

The advantages of the laparoscopic technique are less post-operative pain and speedier recovery from the trivial cuts compared with the incisions several inches long from the older approach. The scars from keyhole surgery are comparable with those of cosmetic surgery, but, to be fair, conventional surgeons are making their incisions considerably smaller and neater (see below). After a laparoscopic cholecystectomy you will be out of hospital in three days and can go back to work when you feel ready, usually within a week. It is reassuring to have virtually unbreakable nylon stitches, and the only restriction is that you must avoid heavy, or more particularly, awkward lifting for three weeks.

Not so long ago it was considered necessary actually to stay in bed for three weeks, but now you can leave hospital in 4–12 days after a traditional cholecystectomy, but after only 2–3 days with a mini-incision. The period before it is wise to go back to work points up

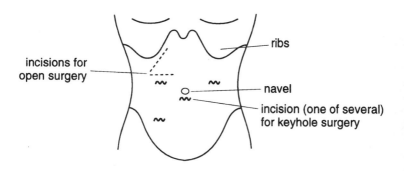

Figure 3 Sites for surgical incision and later scars

the differences between the types of surgery. Against an average of 6.5 days with the laparascopic method, you must allow around 34 days with mini-incision surgery and 5–12 weeks after a standard cholecystectomy. It may seem as though there is no comparison, that the laparoscopic method wins all along the line. However, there are a few snags:

- increased technical difficulty with less room to manoeuvre if something unexpected crops up;
- greater skill, training and practice are required of the surgeon, and this may not be possible in smaller centres;
- although the recovery phase is quick, the operation itself takes longer because it is fiddlier to do. It is no problem for the surgeon to switch to an open operation in midstream should there be any difficulty. For either type of surgery a general anaesthetic is required;
- while well-covered people benefit from having only a few barely noticeable scars in an expanse of flesh, in a thin person the small scars take up a greater proportion of the skin and there is less advantage over having one incision;
- it is more difficult to check for stones in the common bile duct.

X-rays only show radio-opaque stones and can miss many of the common cholesterol type, while ultrasound is less effective with stones outside the gallbladder. To look inside the common bile duct a *choledochoscope* (bile – duct – see) may be introduced through the skin or via an endoscope, a flexible fibreoptic instrument passed down the digestive tract from above.

The risk of there being bile duct stones is higher in these circumstances:

- heart or artery disorders;
- chest problems;
- cirrhosis or other liver disease;
- frailty from advanced age;
- jaundice previously;
- pancreatitis previously;
- an extra-wide cystic duct and common bile duct, a tendency that increases with age;
- large number of small gallbladder stones.

If a small stone slips into the common bile duct it may pass out into the duodenum and finally away with the motions, or it may be extracted through an endoscope.

When you may need a cholecystectomy

- acute cholecystitis, either at the chemical stage or when there is bacterial infection, as in 50 per cent of cases;
- acute emphysematous cholecystitis;
- chronic cholecystitis;
- acute or chronic alcalculous cholecystitis, in which you have the symptoms of cholecystitis, but there are no stones.

The operation may be an *emergency*, for instance in the emphysematous type, *urgent* when there is severe inflammation, or *elective* when there is no special hurry from the clinical point of view, and you and your surgeon can choose, or elect, the time for the operation.

In elective cases, when you may have some weeks to wait, a mild, gradual reduction in your weight, if it is over the odds, puts you in the best possible state for the operation. Aim for a maximum loss of say, 1 lb or 0.45 kg a week. In the few days before the operation, whether you are slim or not-so-slim, you need to go on a low-fat diet – no cream, no fry-ups. Afterwards there are no routine restrictions and most people are back on their normal diet within a few days – but should delay partying.

Miranda

It was 2 a.m. when Miranda was woken up by a terrible pain right across her abdomen and going through to the back. She felt so ill that she thought she was going to die. She wished, now, that she had agreed to have one of those alarms you hang round your neck to call your doctor, an ambulance or the police. But she was a sprightly and independent lady and had pooh-poohed the idea when her daughter had suggested it. At 73 Miranda was not young but not ancient either, and she had managed on her own perfectly well since her husband's death some 10 years ago.

It was shortly after this that she had developed diabetes – the sort that comes in middle age, runs in families and is treated by diet and medicine rather than insulin injections. She had taken that in her stride, and it came as a horrible shock to feel so ill, suddenly, now. She did not know whether she felt freezing cold or too hot and she found herself shaking all over. Miranda realized that she must get help and half-staggered, half-crawled to the telephone. She could not remember the doctor's number but punched in 999. The woman who answered was kind and efficient, asking which service she needed. An ambulance would come to the cottage within 20 minutes, she said, and Miranda should leave all the lights on.

The paramedics took one look at her pale, damp, drawn features and carried her to the ambulance without delay. The surgical registrar was called to Accident and Emergency and found Miranda in a state of shock, in great pain and becoming confused. She kept trying to vomit but all she brought up were strings of bile-stained mucus. An emergency blood count showed that she had a large number of white cells that are poured out to fight infection, but this does not always occur in people of Miranda's age. Her abdomen was acutely tender and felt boggy to the touch. The possibilities were perforated peptic ulcer, acute pancreatitis or heart attack.

Miranda's age and her diabetes made her particularly vulnerable to a fulminant form of inflammation of the gallbladder – emphysematous cholecystitis. It occurs slightly more often in men. A plain X-ray showed gas in Miranda's gallbladder, a dark area, confirming the diagnosis. She would deteriorate rapidly without urgent surgery, but her physical condition had first to be stabilized. Morphine controlled the pain and a saline drip topped up her fluid level and a cephalosporin antibiotic, cefotaxime, was also given through a vein.

Even with the best care emphysematous cholecystitis carries a 20 per cent risk of a fatal outcome. Miranda was one of the 80 per cent who get over this serious illness. She was weak for months afterwards, but had no pain, dyspepsia or other symptoms. By Christmas, six months later, Miranda was back to her old self. Her daughter's gift to her was a personal alarm pendant.

Gallstones and diabetes

Diabetes, added weight and increasing age all have an adverse effect on the working of the gallbladder. An oral cholecystogram shows the gallbladder and its ducts big and slack. It neither fills nor empties efficiently – even after the stimulus of a fatty meal. This means cholestasis, a slowed-down flow of bile and an important factor in stone formation. Diabetics are twice as likely to have gallstones as other people, and the stones are always of the cholesterol type. When a diabetic develops cholecystitis it is likely to be extremely severe, with a tendency to pus formation. Some 20 per cent of those with emphysematous cholecystitis are diabetic.

It cannot be coincidence that the unfortunate Pima Indians of Arizona should not only have the top score for gallstones, but an amazing 50 per cent of them develop the middle-aged type of diabetes even in their twenties. Their traditional diet was fruit and beans and animals they hunted, such as rabbits. Now they live just outside Phoenix, a city of 2.5 million people, have sedentary Western-type jobs and eat a diet based on cheeseburgers, coke and chocolate. We have the same diet and jobs, perhaps accounting for the high prevalence of obesity, gallstones and diabetes in the Western world.

If someone with diabetes has gallstones which are causing no symptoms there is still a strong case for an elective operation to remove the gallbladder. Complications following surgery are more than usually likely in diabetics, but nevertheless most physicians and surgeons consider it worth while to deal with trouble before it happens and rid the patient of the danger of life-threateningly severe cholecystitis. The gallbladder is an organ you will not miss.

The post-cholecystectomy syndrome

Whether incisional or laparoscopic, cholecystectomy is such a safe, well-established operation that the chances are that you will sail through it with nothing worse than a few days' discomfort – and the long-term results are excellent. However there is a 25 per cent risk of running into a mixed bag of symptoms which make up the post-cholecystectomy syndrome. Women are more susceptible than men, especially if they have had gallstone symptoms for five years or more before the operation. Some of those who had been diagnosed as having acalculous (no stones) cholecystitis are among the most vulnerable.

Felicity

Felicity had suffered from mild attacks of biliary colic for some years, at any rate since she was 40, seven years ago. She recovered more or less completely from each bout of symptoms – right-sided pain also affecting her shoulder, and nausea. She also had some symptoms suggesting the irritable bowel syndrome: wind, up and down, bloating and bowels going from one extreme to the other – explosive diarrhoea to obstinate constipation.

X-ray and ultrasound failed to show up any gallstones, but an oral cholecystogram, radionuclide scanning and an intravenous cholangiogram all revealed a large, poorly emptying gallbladder. Its lining was swollen and soggy from an accumulation of fats – cholesterolosis or 'strawberry gallbladder'. It looked red with little yellow flecks of fat, indicating a fault in cholesterol metabolism and is found in 11 per cent of gallbladders that are removed. It happens when there are stones irritating the gallbladder and equally when there are none (acalculous cholecystitis) as in Felicity's case.

Various conditions and events can trigger the latter type, for instance Crohn's disease and the autoimmune disorders such as rheumatoid arthritis. It can also be set off by different forms of injury or trauma, including surgery. In Felicity's case the one relevant event was a severe chip-pan burn some years before. The mechanism linking these problems to the gallbladder remains a mystery, but she was diagnosed as having chronic acalculous cholecystitis.

As the most effective treatment for this or the acute form is removal of the gallbladder, she was booked in for a laparoscopic operation. The procedure went smoothly, but within a few weeks it was clear that she was still experiencing abdominal discomfort, dyspepsia and flatulence – she could not tolerate fatty foods. Her bowels behaved erratically, as they had done previously. This could be due to unrelated irritable bowel syndrome, but these symptoms are often present after a cholecystectomy: one form of the post-cholecystectomy syndrome.

At this stage further investigations were made, but they all proved negative. However, Felicity felt sure that something physical must have been missed and wanted the surgeon to do an exploratory operation, but extra surgery in such cases usually compounds the problem without uncovering any undiagnosed abnormality. Currently Felicity is coping on a low fat diet and antacids, and the situation is to be reviewed in three months. A trial of the alternative therapies is the next step.

Complications and emergency situations: surgical treatment

Cholecystostomy

In some cases of acute cholecystitis the sufferer may be elderly and not strong enough to go through a general anaesthetic and major surgery, yet it is dangerous to do nothing when there is an acutely inflamed gallbladder. Signposts to an urgent operation are:

- a decline in the patient's general condition: they are severely ill;
- signs of peritonitis – inflammation of the lining membrane of the abdomen recognizable by severe pain, tenderness, rigid board-like abdomen and shock;
- pus in the gallbladder or an abscess;
- acute emphysematous cholecystitis (see p. 28).

If the gallbladder is near the front of the abdomen, as it often is in acute inflammation, either mini-incision or laparoscopic cholecystostomy can be performed under a local anaesthetic. Cholecyst*ostomy* means making a hole into the gallbladder, for extracting a stone, releasing pressure and drainage, as opposed to cholecyst*ectomy*, cutting the whole organ out. The cholecystoscope attaches itself to the gallbladder by suction. A stone may simply be taken out, first smashed up by mechanical lithotripsy, or dissolving fluid may be poured over it.

Surgeons are somewhat reluctant to do this operation for two reasons:

1 There is two to three times the risk of immediate serious complications, compared with the situation for cholecystectomy, and a higher mortality. One explanation for this is the age and frailty of the patients for whom this lesser operation is chosen, not the procedure itself.
2 There is a more than 50 per cent likelihood of further trouble with gallstones within the next five years if the gallbladder is left in position. In fact, 60 per cent of those undergoing a cholecystostomy ultimately need to have their gallbladder removed, when they are not so ill.

Raymond

Raymond was nearly 80. For some years he had suffered from a diseased heart valve, and now he had developed an intermittent upset of his heart rhythm – paroxysmal atrial fibrillation. It was at this age and in this situation that his gallbladder became acutely inflamed. Unfortunately, although he looked desperately ill, like many older people, he did not have all the signs and symptoms typical of acute cholecystitis. He did not complain of severe, localized pain, but of a general discomfort of his whole abdomen. When his GP examined him, she found no tenderness or rigidity of the muscles over the gallbladder area, and he had no fever. He had not vomited.

Nevertheless, he was obviously very ill. At the hospital, the surgeon who examined Raymond was able to make out his gallbladder, which he thought was probably full of pus. It was too risky, with his heart condition, to give him a full anaesthetic and a major surgical procedure, so a mini-incision cholecystostomy was performed. There was an abscess in the neck of the gallbladder and a stone lurking in Hartmann's pouch which had probably set the inflammation off. The abscess was drained and the stone removed via the cholecystoscope, and a drainage tube was left in position, to be removed later. Antibiotics were given intravenously (i.e. into a vein), and the cardiologist and the surgical team worked together to bring Raymond through the post-operative period.

Since it seemed unlikely that Raymond would soon, if ever, be fit enough for his gallbladder to be removed, it had to be prevented from causing him further trouble. The cystic duct was quickly obliterated by diathermy, cutting the gallbladder off from the rest of the biliary system. Raymond remains frail, but it is his heart not his gallbladder which is the potential trouble-maker.

Percutaneous gallbladder decompression

This mouthful of syllables means relieving the pressure inside the inflamed gallbladder by passing a hollow needle into it through the skin, under local anaesthetic. Supportive measures must be set up first, specifically intravenous fluids and antibiotics. The infected pus and bile is sucked out and the antibiotic gentamycin instilled into the gallbladder. The drainage tube is left in place for at least ten days, but sedatives and painkillers make this more comfortable. There is a particular risk with acute cholecystitis or empyema (pus-filled gallbladder) of *vaso-vagal* attacks – severe faints – in those with coronary artery disease or other heart problems.

As soon as possible after the acute attack has subsided the stone or stones in the gallbladder must be disposed of by lithotripsy or dissolving them by endoscope. Percutaneous decompression causes less trauma than cholecystostomy but cannot always be performed. It is useful in similar circumstances for someone too infirm for a major procedure.

Fistulas

Fistulas are false passages from one organ to another. Gallstones are responsible for 90 per cent of those in the biliary system, but fistulas only arise in 1 per cent of people with definite gallstone disease. To form a fistula a stone must rub and work its way through the gallbladder wall and whatever is next to it.

Cholecystoduodenal fistula

This type results from a gallstone eroding through the gallbladder and into the duodenum and accounts for 70 per cent of fistulas between the bile system and the intestines. A stone may pass through the new passage into the duodenum and out with the motions, causing no trouble. However, it may get held up lower down in the digestive canal: this is *gallstone ileus*. In three-quarters of cases, obstruction of the intestines due to a gallstone affects the last part of the small intestine, the ileum. This is also the part most susceptible to Crohn's disease, which itself makes the passage through the gut narrower. Only 15 per cent of stones lodge in the jejunum, the upper part of the small intestine, while 10 per cent get no further than the duodenum and another 10 per cent reach the sigmoid colon, near the very end of the digestive tract. In the last case it is usually associated with diverticular disease, a wear-and-tear phenomenon in which little pockets form in the colon wall and can easily trap a stone.

Air shows up in half the X-rays when there is obstruction, and a calcified stone will also be visible. Typically this will be seen to change its location in a series of X-rays, accompanied by a change in the symptoms. A barium 'meal', opaque to X-ray, or a CT scan may help with the diagnosis.

Clinical signs and symptoms of intestinal obstruction, as in gallstone ileus:

- colicky pain accompanied by gurgles in the abdomen (borbor-ygmi);

- vomiting if the obstruction is high up in the intestines, but it may not occur if the colon is the part affected;
- bloating: this may be generalized or confined to a particular area;
- bowel movements: in high obstruction there is no immediate effect, but complete obstruction low down means that nothing is passed through the back passage, not even gas.

The doctor's examination is vital for the diagnosis, backed up by X-rays or other investigations if necessary. Obstruction may be complete or incomplete, acute or chronic, intermittent or constant.

Management begins with supportive treatment and intravenous fluids, but as soon as the clinical state is stable urgent surgery is started, mainly a matter of repair.

Enterotomy

This is the simplest operation and most suitable for the old and sick, who are likely to be the people concerned. It involves a small cut in the abdomen to examine the situation and put the anatomy to rights, so that the fistula is no longer open. This is also a chance to check for other stones in the intestines or gallbladder – they are a cause of recurrence in some 5 per cent of cases. If the symptoms do not improve markedly after enterotomy, an ERCP (see p. 57) is a further check.

Cholecystocolic fistula

This is caused by a stone working its way from the gallbladder directly into the colon. The result is profuse diarrhoea because of the irritating effects of the bile acids. Plain X-rays may show air in the gallbladder and a barium enema will clarify the situation at the colon end. ERCP may also be useful.

Operation: cholecystectomy and closure of the fistula.

Cholecystocholedochal fistula (gallbladder to common bile duct)

This fistula usually develops from Mirizzi's syndrome (see p. 31) in which a gallstone in the gallbladder presses against the gallbladder wall and erodes a passage into the common bile duct.

Treatment: simple cholecystectomy is the chosen treatment in most cases, but sometimes part of the gallbladder wall is used to repair the gap in the bile duct wall.

Choledocholithotomy

Bile duct stones are usually dealt with through an endoscope or by the percutaneous method, through the skin.

In some cases surgery is preferable:

- bile duct stones found during elective, conventional removal of the gallbladder but not in the case of high-risk patients or older people who could not withstand the operation being prolonged;
- stones found during an emergency cholecystectomy for complicated disease, including cholecystocholedochal fistula (gallbladder to common bile duct);
- resolving mild inflammation of any bile duct (cholangitis);
- resolving acute pancreatitis;
- stone in the part of the bile duct system within the liver;
- failure of non-surgical methods of removing bile duct stones.

Premalignant conditions

These give a warning of the danger of cancer of the gallbladder developing and allow for preventive surgery.

- 'porcelain gallbladder', in which there are excessive deposits of calcium in its wall;
- xanthogranulomatous cholecystitis: sometimes the bile pigments penetrate the connective tissue of the gallbladder and cause marked inflammation, with disturbance of the local fat metabolism.

Treatment in both cases: cholecystectomy, removing the organ that is in danger.

Cancer of the gallbladder

This is an uncommon tumour, especially in men. The peak age for its starting up is 70–75 years. It is almost invariably associated with gallstones and arises in the mucous membrane lining the gallbladder where it produces extra mucus. Sometimes it presents with the symptoms of acute inflammation of the gallbladder or empyema. It is for this reason that a biopsy (microscopic examination of a tiny sample of tissue) is always made at a gallbladder operation, including cholecystectomy.

Operations: removal of part of the bed of the gallbladder at the same time as the cholecystectomy has been shown to be beneficial in some cases of cancer, but in others a bypass operation, isolating the gallbladder is the best answer.

Nutrition is of great importance as weight loss is one of the main symptoms. Intravenous nourishment provides a quick and easy boost to the weight, before settling down to a build-up diet.

TREATMENT 2: SURGICAL

Chemotherapy and radiotherapy: the jury is still out about their value in this disorder.

10

The alternatives 1: self-help

If you have a clear-cut problem, such as a gallstone lodged in the common bile duct, causing pain and jaundice, medicines and surgical procedures can be wonderfully effective – sometimes even life-saving. If a particular enemy bug has set up an infection in your gallbladder, the right antibiotic will zap it. It is useful to know what your doctor is talking about and if he or she suggests some medication, what it is supposed to do. It is useful too, at least to have heard of some of the medical procedures and surgical operations and to understand what some of the jaw-breaking terms mean. But you are not just a body with gallstones getting in the mechanism, to be put right like a faulty automobile.

What if your pains and other symptoms do not respond to the doctor's treatment? Or a raft of tests and investigations throw up negative results and your doctor tells you happily 'There's nothing wrong', yet you know that you do not feel right.

This is the time to consider what else is on offer. If straight medicine cannot help or leaves you only a little better, there is no need to despair. Fortunately there is a wide choice of 'alternative' therapies; they are called 'complementary', if you use them as an add-on to the conventional treatment rather than instead. A totally different approach may be just what you need. For starters, instead of being regarded as 'that case of chronic cholecystitis', in need of the right drug or operation, alternative therapists treat you as an individual with fears and feelings as well as symptoms, and a very human need for comfort and reassurance when you are suffering.

Alternative therapies, because they are not scientifically cut-and-dried always contain an element of hope, a glimpse of the light at the end of the weary tunnel of illness. Another advantage is that, rather than being the passive recipient of what the expert thinks best, you are personally involved in the decisions and the treatment. It must surely work better if this is in harmony with your wishes and feelings, with the therapist helping you to find your chosen way to health. Alternative therapies aim at strengthening your own mental and physical defences, not primarily at killing hostile germs, destroying gallstones or blanking out the symptoms.

Of course, there are disadvantages when you take the alternative route. You will not get the dramatic 'cures' that the medical model may produce, for example the instant relief from gallstone pain with shock-wave lithotripsy. On the other hand, you do not risk the complications that can arise with surgery or some other procedures, nor the side-effects which are the bugbear of using powerful drugs. A disadvantage that has a silver lining is that no alternative therapy is free, whether it is a herbal medicine you buy over the counter, or the skill of the therapist whom you have picked. With a simple purchase you have made a voluntary investment, a positive start, and when a therapist is involved, by your paying him or her a fee personally you are demonstrating that he or she is the person you want and whom you believe is worth it. This is a fine basis for working together.

There is a bewildering number of alternative therapies to choose from and they come in four basic packs:

- self-help, including self-help in a group;
- therapies requiring the skill of an operator, for instance, a reflexologist or hypnotist;
- those in which you need someone to show you the ropes, or teach you the technique, to enable you are to practise it on your own. Diet is one example and acupressure another;
- herbal medicines – you can buy these in a health store and the larger chemists' shops often have a section devoted to alternative medicines, lotions and potions.

A dash of faith comes into all these therapies, whether medicines or manipulation. In alternative medicine there are rarely any double-blind, placebo-controlled, clinical trials with statistics to prove their efficacy as in standard medicine, so you rely on the personal recommendation of other people (their number is not even counted), based on their own experience. You could be one of those who benefit, perhaps miraculously.

There are some provisos on using these methods:

1 Pain: if you have very severe pain or are seized with sudden acute pain such as can grip you in acute appendicitis or acute cholecystitis, for safety's sake you must go straight for standard medical help: pharmaceutical painkillers and surgery if necessary. Alternative treatments are not geared to emergencies. They are gentle and slow-acting and can only deal with ongoing conditions, not for instance with a burst gallbladder (this is in fact

a rarity). It is the chronic symptoms and nagging problems which respond best to alternative therapies.

2 Side-effects: there is no guarantee that herbal medicines, just because they come from natural sources, are harmless. Think of Deadly Nightshade, a modest little plant. Some of the herbs that are used are very potent, and can produce unwanted results, especially if you happen to be sensitive to one of the ingredients. In November 1999 the Committee on the Safety of Medicines contacted all the doctors in the UK notifying them of ill-effects, some fatal, of certain traditional Chinese medicines and some from the Indian subcontinent. They are asking doctors here to report any serious adverse reactions to herbal medicines. This brings them into line with the ordinary pharmaceutical products.

Quite apart from medical disasters, pain is the symptom which overrides all others in importance and demands attention. Your body, your brain – the organ of the mind, and your emotions, are all part of the whole that is you. Pain reflects this. It is experienced in the brain – proof is in the effect of an anaesthetic, which knocks out your brain temporarily and you feel nothing even when a surgeon is removing your gallbladder. The pain your brain registers, refers, as a rule, to some other part of your body, from your big toe to your bile duct. Your emotions influence how much you feel the pain and how much it distresses you. A footballer who has received a nasty hack on the shin from an opponent's boot may be quite unaware of the injury in the excitement of the game. On the other hand, if you are already anxious, any pain feels sharper, or you are even more restless when you are depressed.

It makes sense to approach the problem of pain on a broad front. Our instinct is to focus on the physical aspect, but it works better when the mental and emotional facets are also considered. Whatever method you choose to deal with your pain, first you need to assess your stress level, and then try to reduce it.

Life-events: run through everything that has happened to you in the last six months, and list anything that disrupted your lifestyle or altered your outlook in some way. You may have gone through a bereavement, failed an examination or been burgled, or had ongoing niggling worries – about money, the kids, the computer going down and the washing machine packing up. These are stressors. There are also desirable events such as getting married or starting a new business which send your world topsy-turvy. These hype up your stress level just as much.

How can you measure your stress status? What to look out for:

- feeling on edge;
- difficulty in concentrating;
- disturbed sleep;
- restless but achieving nothing – cannot relax;
- tired but alert: your eyes feel prickly;
- snappy to other people.

It is understandable that in this state you just cannot cope with pain – it feels a thousand times worse. Other symptoms, too, such as nausea, headache or loss of appetite (or the reverse, compulsive eating) are worse too.

Reducing your stress level is an essential preliminary to treatment. To do so:

- Identify the causes of your stress and take practical steps to ease them.
- Breathing exercises, to do twice a day and when stressed: breathe in all the way, quickly, through your nose, then breathe out as slowly as possible and practise this. Aim at 2 seconds breathing in, 8 seconds breathing out. Go on repeating this for 5–10 minutes. You can use this when you feel tension or pain building up.
- Muscular relaxation: there are several different systems for this (see below) but it can be as simple as lying on your back with a small pillow under your head, trying to imagine that you are in a warm bath. You feel your muscles relaxing in turn, starting from the toes. Go through this up to ten times.
- Visualization, to follow on from relaxation: you are lying on a beach, watching the clouds drift by and the seagulls whirling and swooping, and listening to the slow rhythm of the sea. Or you are walking through a meadow with big daisies and poppies and other wild plants bending in the breeze – or a hundred other scenes of peace and beauty in nature. This is the equivalent of the Vedas' cure for stress – just sitting still.

Anne

Anne was 36 and she was stressed out with a part-time job, the kids, the house and a husband who worked all hours. She had been getting attacks of pain on the right side of her abdomen, creeping round to the back, and she felt sick with it. She had not got a helicobacter infection, so her doctor suspected a 'grumbling gallbladder'. He said that she was rather young, but nowadays women in particular were getting gallstone trouble earlier and earlier. The children, aged two and three, had just got over chickenpox and were still whiny and demanding. Anne had been too distracted for the past few weeks to eat a proper meal herself, but had daylong nibbles of cholesterol-laden cheese, chocolate and sweet biscuits – and coffee.

Her pain became more persistent and when she found herself biting everyone's head off she decided to do something about it. As a kick-off she had a 12-hour mini-fast, drinking only non-fizzy water and fruit juice. Then she started having regular, sit-down meals with the emphasis on whole foods, fruit and vegetables. She felt more comfortable wearing loose-fitting gear, which was suitable for the stress-reducing ploy of progressive relaxation exercises – 10 minutes a day – and in spare moments pressing the acupressure points on her face. She had heard that this relieved the stress component of stomachache. The other points ran down in two parallel lines from the breastbone halfway to the navel. When she felt nauseated she pressed the points on the front of her wrist, but decided against buying an elastic wristband with a pad at the front, intended to provide continuous pressure. The health store assistant said that it was not really firm enough compared with finger pressure.

Anne also treated herself to some essential oils used in aromatherapy to make her warm baths really therapeutic – using five drops of each oil directly in the water. Scots pine was the one recommended for gallbladder pain and she also chose jasmine and lemon, for general stress. As soon as she had started on her personal self-help course Anne's mood became more positive. She was more relaxed with the children and they in turn were less of a handful. The big test will be whether she has fewer attacks of gallbladder pain over the next few months.

Self-help

There is no shame in having help when you need it, but it is very satisfying and a boost to the confidence if you can manage to do some effective therapy by yourself. In some cases it is almost instinctual: for example, the time-honoured hot water bottle, nowadays gel-filled or an electric pad, put on your abdomen where it hurts, or slow deep breathing to calm yourself. In other cases written instructions in a book are enough. For a large group of valuable treatments, however, you need a few sessions from a qualified therapist before you can take over confidently.

Relaxation methods

There is simple relaxation, as described in the preliminary stress-reduction package, and more structured types. The most effective are three which are much the same: *sequential muscle relaxation* (*SMR*), *progressive relaxation* and *Jacobson relaxation*. They all reduce mental as well as physical tension and take the edge off pain.

Ernest

Ernest swears by SMR. When he feels the first twinge, possibly a gallstone on the move, or anxiety-driven muscle spasm, he swings into a session of relaxation. Sitting comfortably in a chair in a dark room, he tenses a group of muscles, for instance those of his right forearm, holds the tension for a count of 15, then releases it gently while breathing out. After 10–15 seconds' pause he repeats the process with another set of muscles, continuing until he has worked through his whole body. Next he combines two and then three sets of muscles together. The whole exercise takes him 15–30 minutes, and at the end of it his body is relaxed and his mind calm. Usually he repeats it daily for a couple of weeks – longer would be better.

The Mitchell method of relaxation is slightly different. Lying on your back, legs apart, arms outstretched and fingers spread, you take up as much floor space as possible, moving each part of you, and holding each new position. Then lie on your front and bend your back into an arc – any position is all right so long as it is not one you would use if you were anxious or upset. In that case you might curl into the foetal attitude, hugging yourself and clenching your fists.

Relaxation classes are often included in straight medicine as an extra, typically in a course of six or eight weekly sessions, each lasting an hour or so, to be accompanied by daily sessions on your own of 15–30 minutes. These should continue after the course is finished; indeed, some people with no health problems find them helpful in conserving their mental and physical energy. Unlike powerful medicines, most alternative therapies take weeks or a few months before you feel their effects fully. The short cut of taking tablets to help you relax and douse out pain often does not pay. You can get caught up in a vicious spiral of increasing doses of tranquillizers to relax you and painkillers to dull the pain.

Both these classes of drugs are depressants and their efficacy declines with use. Worse than that, your spirits will inevitably sink and you end up with your symptoms breaking through, plus a load of side-effects: headache, dizziness, fatigue, and stomach or bowel disturbances. These increase inexorably with the dosage.

Self-help groups

With relaxation therapies the precise diagnosis is irrelevant. They have a non-specific beneficial effect on long-term pain. The social aspect of attending relaxation classes is meeting other people – this is a plus. Pain can be lonely, so it is a relief to share it with other sufferers, in a group who will not be bored or irritated by hearing of your day-to-day experience of it. Some GPs arrange self-help groups for a mixed bag of patients with pain – from arthritis or migraine to gallstones playing up.

Physical exercise

Walking, dancing, free-standing exercises, and videos (mainly for slimmers) may all help you to relax. The special types like yoga are described in Chapter 11. Anything too vigorous, however, can make your pain worse. The distraction component of exercise, as with the other relaxation techniques, serves to keep your mind from dwelling on the pain or other symptoms. For your general health it is as important as sleep and nourishment.

Autogenic training

This is a technique for gaining some control over the degree of tension in your muscles (responsible for how much you feel pain), and also the circulation to various parts. It is often taught, but you can try it out on your own.

1 Lie on your bed or carpeted floor with a small pillow. Let your knees bend slightly if that feels more comfortable. Close your eyes.
2 Concentrate on your right hand and arm and tell yourself silently that they feel heavy. If you have a helper they will say the words aloud.
3 Imagine your arm so relaxed and loose and heavy that it is

beginning to sink down into the bed. Think of its weight. Try to keep focusing on its weight, its heaviness – it would be too heavy to lift. For a full minute keep reminding yourself, over and over, that your hand and arm are limp and weighty. It is difficult to keep this up – everyone finds it so – so do not expect to crack it first time. When you do succeed you will feel a pleasant sense of release.

4 Now focus on your left hand and arm and go through the same exercise, also for a full minute.

5 Next concentrate on your left leg, then your right leg, with a good minute on each.

6 Go back to your right arm and hand and tell yourself that they are feeling particularly warm. Hold this thought for another minute.

7 Go through the same process with your left arm and hand, left leg and then right leg. When you feel the warmth stay with it, enjoy it and let it spread through you, including the gallbladder area.

8 Concentrate on your forehead. Silently affirm that it feels cool and refreshed. Repeat this message and hold it.

The whole exercise takes only 10–15 minutes. Repeat it once or twice a day and you will find it easier and easier to induce the sensations of heaviness, warmth and coolness. Achieving heaviness means deep relaxation, and warmth and coolness show some control over your circulation.

Self-hypnosis is next cousin to autogenic training. It is better termed *autosuggestion*. It was over a century ago that a French chemist turned hypnotist, Emile Coué, found that if his patients repeated to themselves 15–20 times, night and morning: 'Every day in every way I am getting better and better', it helped some of those with seemingly hopeless problems, including chronic pain. Talking to a mirror was the best way.

Louise Hay, a present-day therapist in America, recommends a kind of reverse Couéism. She helps her clients to understand the detrimental effects of negative thoughts, and they have to set up a mental barrier to them, by repetition.

Directed visualization

This follows on naturally from relaxation and the simple visualization of safe, harmonious or uplifting natural scenes which have the aim of inducing a sense of contentment. Only when you have achieved this, direct your mind to the area of your pain. Now picture the pain itself:

- sharp and stabbing – imagine it as sharp icicles, now melting in the rays of the sun;
- colicky – think of evil gnomes taking turns twisting your flesh; to get rid of them there is a rescue squad from your body's defence organization who will drive them away;
- boring – a bad giant with a corkscrew who will lose all his strength when his hair is cut, like Samson, but by a good angel;
- or pain may just appear in your mind's eye as all over red, but you, by taking thought, can make the colour gradually fade to pink and then white.

'The liver flush'

This is something you can try yourself when you are weary with a nagging gallbladder ache. It is a tonic for your biliary system with a reputation for seeing off gallstones. Start by applying a hot pack – a small towel wrung out in hot water – to the place where it hurts in the front and another to your back, and leave them on for 15 minutes. Sip peppermint water while you wait. For six days eat only wholefoods and apples, with apple juice to drink, no tea or coffee.

On the morning of the seventh day drink a small cupful of olive oil and lemon juice, half-and-half. This stimulates your liver to pour out a good flow of bile which helps to dissolve gallstones and wash the small ones out of your system. Go back to your usual diet but miss out animal fats, fizzy drinks and caffeine.

Foot massage

It needs an expert to apply reflexology but gently rubbing, stroking and kneading the sides and soles of your feet is oddly comforting. Pressing your thumb into the centre of the arch on the sole of your right foot for 10–15 seconds is said to link up with your gallbladder and switch off any pain.

Aromatherapy

This also involves massage and is another healing process for which you require the help of a trained therapist, but you can get some of the benefits yourself by putting the appropriate essential oils into your bath water, as Anne did, or vaporizing them on a burner. Scots pine is the top recommendation for gallstone pain. Rubbing a mix of marjoram and rosemary oils, ten drops each, with five drops of black pepper oil in a carrier oil into your skin (see directions on bottle) is a mini-treatment you can give yourself.

Acupressure

This gives some of the pain relief provided by acupuncture. The places to apply firm finger pressure for gallbladder trouble are three fingers width away from each side of the navel, or the pressure points that Anne used, halfway down to the navel level from the breastbone. You will be able to tell which of these is best for you. A neat trick by which you can keep up the pressure longer than with your finger is to lie on your stomach with a tennis ball underneath you just below the ribs on the right. The facial acupressure points which Anne used for reducing stress are just below nose level, vertically down from your eyes.

Meditation

Healing through mind over matter is most effective if all extraneous thoughts and worries are put aside. Meditation is different from daydreaming, which inevitably allows your anxieties to come to the surface. It is described, confusingly, as *passive concentration* and also as *active attention*. The essence is to clear your mind of everyday clutter and concentrate on a single word which you repeat. This is called a mantra, and you can choose any word you like. Some people prefer to focus on a mental picture, while others find a lighted candle the easiest to fix their mind on. Before you can start meditating you need to feel physically relaxed, sitting calm and still, and then get your mind into similar mode.

Meditation damps down stress and pain and induces a sense of peace and tranquillity. The brainwaves slip into a particular rhythm which is neither that of sleep nor normal wakefulness: an electroencephalogram demonstrates this. At this stage your blood pressure switches to a lower level, and other physiological activities such as muscle tone and the production of stomach acid all operate at a maintenance rate.

TM, transcendental meditation, became extremely popular in the 1970s, not necessarily for people with definite problems but as an aid to keeping their mental equilibrium with whatever life might throw at them. Anyone can meditate, but TM is best taught by a guru since its roots are in Eastern philosophy. Statues of Buddha are often in an attitude of peaceful meditation, sometimes in the lotus position, but also reclining or leaning on one elbow.

Crystal healing

This is another unproven therapy which has become fashionable, although it has a long history. The theory is that different crystals and semi-precious stones can influence, by physical contact, a person's spiritual state or mood. There are lists of mood and personality problems indicating which stone is thought to be most appropriate. A small locket, worn round the neck, contains the chosen stone.

There seems to be no scientific reason for a stone to have any effect, but it is certainly harmless and rather pleasant to wear a piece of jewellery like a good-health amulet, such as the ancient Egyptians employed.

The placebo effect is powerful. It is well known to doctors when they are trying a new or different medicine on their patient. The sufferer is likely to feel better almost at once, but the snag with the placebo effect is that it fades after about three weeks.

Bach Flower Remedies

Dr Edward Bach brought out his flower theory in the 1920s and it caught on at once. Like Louise Hay (see p. 90) he was convinced that ugly and negative thoughts and attitudes affected emotional and bodily well-being, life events (difficult to understand how) and the ability to withstand misfortune. He developed 38 flower and tree remedies, since expanded to more than a hundred, each geared to fit the individual's personality and current psychological state rather than his or her symptom or illness. These medicines are 'essences' or simple extracts of the plants, and they are intended to relieve painful conditions caused by an underlying emotional state. It may sound far-fetched, but like crystal healing it can do no harm and is a pleasant, even beautiful idea. Flower remedies are used all over the world by thousands of people who believe they are beneficial. Fifty firms produce them.

Many modern medicines, for instance Taxol, the new treatment for cancer of the ovary, are derived from plants – in this case the yew tree. Dr Bach's cures may, by chance, have a beneficial chemical effect. Some of the flowers and plants and what they are said to do:

- impatiens – encourages patience;
- mimulus – gives courage to the faint-hearted;

- elm – restores confidence when you have felt overwhelmed;
- clematis – aids concentration;
- chestnut bud – helps you to learn from experience;
- sweet chestnut – gives hope in a state of despair;
- olive – regenerates mental peace and balance lost through overwork;
- wild rose – recreates lost motivation.

According to the theory that your mental state can make you vulnerable physically, you pick your medicine according to your emotional needs. Bach's Rescue Remedy is for use in extreme stress and disaster. It contains five ingredients:

- rock rose for anxiety and panic;
- cherry plum for loss of control;
- Star of Bethlehem for shock and trauma;
- clematis to focus the mind;
- impatiens – as above.

Electromagnetic therapy

This is a direct attack on pain. Small magnets are held against the skin by sticking plaster, or sometimes sewn into the clothes in the area where there is pain.

There are many more healing therapies, some steeped in folklore, others with a long respectable history. What is certain is that a scientific explanation will ultimately be found for many of them, and meanwhile, if you derive benefit from one of them, use it now. Do not wait for proof and do not feel ashamed.

11

The alternatives 2: help from a therapist

Pain is private and personal, more so than any other symptom of something being wrong. Nobody else can see or feel your pain, nausea or fatigue and it is a bleak burden to carry on your own. If you tell your friends, family or colleagues they will be sympathetic to start with, but quickly become bored and irritated with hearing about your anxieties and how you are feeling physically. Your family doctor is 'rushed off his or her feet' and consultations average out at three minutes each – just time to write a scrip, or refer you to a surgeon, but no time to talk through your feelings, fears, hopes and wishes.

It is in this situation that complementary therapy has blossomed, becoming increasingly popular since the 1980s. Today it is accepted as filling a gaping hole in the care provided by traditional medicine. The holistic approach means encompassing the whole person and this may involve an orthodox and a complementary practitioner working side by side. More and more, 'alternative' has become 'complementary'.

While you can help yourself to a certain extent, it is of tremendous value to have the guidance and encouragement of an experienced therapist, even with the simpler forms of treatment. There is an abundance of disparate therapies and therapists and your first hurdle is to find a therapist to suit you. What they all have in common is a belief held by both the Chinese and the ancient Greeks – that the body has remarkable powers of self-healing and the practitioner's role is to release and enhance them. This basic aim of the alternative therapies is often neglected by conventional medicine.

When you are choosing your therapist, it is reassuring to have a personal recommendation from someone you know, or to learn that the therapist is attached to one of the reputable alternative medicine organizations. You will need a preliminary discussion before committing yourself financially or time-wise to a course of treatment, unlike signing up with a GP. You will be asked to outline your problems and the type of help you hope to get. In return you will want to know what treatments are available, which one the therapist recommends and how the chances of your full recovery are rated. One of the important factors in deciding on a specific treatment is your personal preference.

Guidelines for choosing a therapist

- If you do not want to talk about your private life and personal details, avoid homoeopathy and psychotherapy, and go for aromatherapy or reflexology.
- If you do not like needles, give acupuncture a miss. Try acupressure or shiatsu.
- If you do not want to take your clothes off, do not have a full massage, go for yoga or the Alexander technique.

Massage

Pressing or rubbing where it hurts is instinctive, and massage is a form of medical care that goes back to the earliest civilizations. Egyptian tomb paintings depict it and the time-hallowed Indian and Chinese medical manuscripts mention it. For the Greeks and Romans it was the principal treatment for pain. The writings of Hippocrates, around 500 BC, include this passage: 'The physician must be experienced in many things, but assuredly in rubbing.' Julius Caesar, half a millennium later, had daily massage for his neuralgia.

The type we use today, Swedish massage, was devised by Per Ling in the 1890s as a treatment for all bodily ills, but especially pain. The goal was to achieve mental and physical 'calmness and wholeness'. A full body massage takes about an hour and is an agreeable experience – soothing, relaxing and making you feel cared for. Pain loses its edge, in the gallbladder as elsewhere.

There are several modifications of straightforward massage.

Aromatherapy

The ancient Greeks took scented baths before rubbing oil into their bodies. Aromatherapy is a massage using various essential oils from plants, with carrier oils. The aroma is pleasant, but it is also thought that the oils absorbed through the skin and by inhalation (check directions on bottles) have specific medical effects. For all gallbladder complaints Scots pine is recommended. For indigestion and flatulence, rosemary, peppermint and clary sage may help. Nervous tension is eased away best by orange and sandalwood.

Reflexology

Foot massage, or reflexology, is another form used by the ancients, and in 1915 Dr William Fitzgerald adapted the Chinese idea of energy zones represented by specific points in the body, for instance on the ear, into a theory that the whole body is mapped out on the soles of the feet. Having your feet massaged is remarkably pleasant and certainly harmless. It is said to work especially well in disorders of the internal organs, such as the biliary system, where there is a stress component. The liver is linked to a broad band on the sole, just below the arch of the foot, with the gallbladder in the middle and the shoulder next to it.

Biodynamic massage

Gerda Boyasen, a Norwegian psychologist and physiotherapist, combined her two skills into a massage therapy which aims to release energy bound up in the digestive organs and causing pain. Bowel gurgles are believed to indicate success.

Healing and touch

It is natural to put your arm round somebody in pain or distress, and holding hands in the dark infuses courage into a small child. The 'laying on of hands' which takes place still in some churches is meant to heal physical as well as spiritual problems.

The therapeutic touch (TT)

This is a term used most often in the United States. Dolores Krieger, a Professor of Nursing, popularized this ancient practice in the 1970s. It involves the transfer of life force or healing energy from one person to another, supposedly. What has been scientifically demonstrated is that the effects of stress on the immune system are reduced by TT. It involves nothing more dangerous than a light touch, and sometimes not even that. The healer's thoughts alone are considered by some therapists to be enough. The hands are held close to, but not in actual contact with the subject as he or she concentrates.

Reiki is a newer variation from Japan, said to be derived from a treatment used in the Tibetan monasteries. It is said to bring about what is 'the highest good', not necessarily the cure requested by the sufferer.

Healing used to be called 'faith healing' and, as with all therapies, including the placebo, belief in its power enhances the effect. There has been a string of remarkable results involving healers. The personality and commitment of the healer are paramount, but honesty and plausibility do not necessarily coincide.

Movement therapies

Yoga

This is the best known of the mind/body techniques, an oriental art in movement that has been practised for hundreds of years. It is said to be the antidote to stress, both physical and mental. It consists of slow, deliberate movements leading to various positions of the body. The Pose of Tranquillity is the one intended to benefit the stomach and liver: you lie on your back and, while breathing in, swing your legs up and over so that your knees are above your face. You keep your balance with your hands and arms. The Salute to the Sun is the yoga beginner's exercise:

- while standing, raise your arms above your head, lean forwards slightly and bend your knees;
- bend forward smoothly, until your chest touches your thighs. Drop your arms behind your calves;
- return to the standing position with your arms high and your knees still slightly bent. Arch your back.

Then repeat. Ideally you should do an hour's yoga exercises every day. Half that is a realistic minimum. This was a very simple exercise, but to go further you need to learn from an expert. Some of the poses, apart from being complicated to achieve, can, for instance put an undue strain on your neck or other parts. My son-in-law, demonstrating a yoga exercise he had just learned, found himself unable to get out of a painful position – without help.

Tai chi

This movement system is so highly regarded in China that it is not uncommon to see large groups of people practising it in the public parks. The movements are gentler, slower and more harmonious than those of yoga, and it is especially helpful when physical and emotional suffering are intertwined. Its object is to enhance *chi*, the life force.

The Alexander technique

This was evolved by an actor early in the twentieth century to improve his posture and breathing. He found it made him and others who used the technique feel fitter in every way. Four to six lessons are necessary to learn the method: the teacher uses a hands-on approach to help you get into the correct bodily postures.

Deep massage techniques

Rolfing is a vigorous type of deep massage in which the practitioner uses his or her hands, fingers, knuckles and elbows with considerable pressure. The patient's breathing must synchronize with the massage. Self-help exercises, known as movement integration, follow the session. This treatment is a catch-all stimulant, relaxant and tranquillizer.

Hellerwork, similar to Rolfing, is a form of deep pressure massage. It is sold in a package of 11 90-minute sessions.

Tragerwork is a massage technique geared to reducing muscle tension and is combined with mentastatics to reduce mental stress. Any of these may make pain worse.

The Feldenkrais method, another massage method, is distinguished by having been invented by an Israeli atomic physicist.

None of these therapies is useful specifically for gallstone troubles.

Acupuncture

This is the prince of pain treatments and, because it works so well for that, it has also been tried, with variable success, for other symptoms. It is usually successful with abdominal pain and discomfort. Acupuncture was practised in China 3,500 years ago and stone acupuncture needles have been found in Inner Mongolia. Today the needles are of gold, silver or steel and so fine that you may not feel them being inserted.

Acupuncture is in routine use in pain clinics in the West now. It is thought that it works by interrupting pain messages to the brain, and either distracting it or stimulating the production of endorphins, the body's own morphine analogues. There are complex, finely detailed maps showing lines of force, the meridians, and hundreds of acupuncture points, each connected with a particular part of the body, including the gallbladder. Two important meridians relate to the liver and stomach. Two forces, yin and yang, need to be in balance for the body to be in good health, and the interaction between them is thought to produce *chi*, the life force.

Hari

Hari at 37 suffered from cholangitis, inflammation of bile ducts within the liver, associated with infection and brown pigment stones. He was often conscious of a dull ache in his abdomen and he had not felt really well for months. His doctor suggested acupuncture as surgery had nothing to offer and courses of antibiotics were having less and less effect. Hari's acupuncturist had been trained by a Chinese expert, but he did not enjoy the sessions although it was discomfort rather than pain that he experienced.

They lasted 30–90 minutes, the longest at the beginning. He had weekly sessions and expected to have 15 or 20 of them. The therapist asked him about ordinary day-to-day happenings, his work, his wife, their leisure times. Over the four months' treatment he found himself gradually feeling happier, stronger and more able to put up with the pain, which was now less severe.

Electro-acupuncture involves passing a small current through the acupuncture needles, but the twisting of the needles in the traditional way is equally effective.

Osteopathy and chiropractic

These are both hands-on manipulative therapies. In the past, chiropractic in particular was seen as a complete treatment for physical disorders, all of which were thought to be due to misalignment of the small bones of the spine. Nowadays they are generally regarded as related to physiotherapy and good for muscle and joint pain only.

Hypnosis

This is the ultimate in relaxation. It involves a therapist, a hypnotist, inducing a deeply relaxed state called a 'hypnotic trance', during which you are likely to take on board, uncritically, any ideas he may suggest to you. Of course these are likely only to be about the pain in your gallbladder fading or being replaced by a warm glow, but because you are putting yourself in a vulnerable position it is essential to check out the qualifications of your hypnotist. He or she should be associated with the British Society of Medical and Dental Hypnosis or the National College of Hypnosis and Psychotherapy.

Post-hypnotic suggestion applies to your thinking, feeling and behaviour after the session, for instance that you will find it easy to use self-hypnosis for relaxation and the dulling of pain.

Electronic apparatus

Biofeedback

In the 1930s electronic devices were being developed to detect minute physical changes in the body, and by the 1980s stress management courses using biofeedback were up and running. Skin temperature, sweating, muscle tension, brainwaves, blood pressure and heart rate can all be monitored and shown on a VDU. You need at least six half-hour sessions with the machine to begin to gain some control over your body's responses to stress.

Successful stress management is shown by warm skin, little sweating, a slow, even heart rate and brainwave rhythm – and you feel better in yourself, with less pain and less anxiety about it.

TENS

TENS is transcutaneous electrical nerve stimulation, and is a method of blocking the pain messages from a particular area. TENS is risk-free and side-effect-free. It is used in all pain clinics, as a first choice, and it is also possible to buy a TENS machine. They cost £50–150, but there is no great advantage in the more expensive models.

Shelley

Shelley is a sceptic, and she did not believe this little machine could help her, but she agreed to give it a whirl. Two small pads were attached to her skin, one immediately over a tender place, the other just to the side of the area of pain – thought to be from chronic cholecystitis. A smear of gel under each pad improved the electrical contact. When the apparatus was switched on a mild electrical current passed between them. Shelley was told to increase its intensity herself until she felt a pleasant tingling sensation which replaced the nagging pain.

She was surprised, and even more pleased, when the effect continued for many hours after the treatment. She found it increasingly helpful with further sessions and had no side-effects.

Intasound is treatment by sound waves. The apparatus is hand-held in the area where there is pain, and silent sound waves passing through the tissues may reduce any pain.

Creative arts

Painting, modelling, dance and music all serve to enrich your life. They take your mind away from minor pains, nausea and everyday troubles, on the wings of imagination. Only we humans have this outlet.

Most alternative therapy has no direct effect on definite physical problems, but from its holistic approach can make you feel more at peace and focused less on your symptoms. However, it is essential when you have sudden or severe pain, vomiting or the merest hint of jaundice, that you check in with a medical practitioner before anything else. Sometimes people who are enthusiastic supporters of alternative medicine feel guilty that they cannot manage without conventional treatment.

The sensible course is to take the best of both worlds and make the alternative therapy complementary.

12

Herbal medicine and homoeopathy

Herbal medicines

Ayurveda

Ayurveda, 'the science of life', is a system of medicine that has been in use in India for the last 4,500 years. It includes a range of herbal remedies, but most of these have not been fully evaluated. Some of them are powerful purgatives, also enemas, but neither of these is to be recommended, and there have been recent reports of unfortunate side-effects from some of the lesser-known preparations. Two well-tried, harmless recipes which are said to benefit digestive problems are grated fresh ginger in tea or milk, and ripe banana with cumin. The latter also helps with sleep.

TCM, traditional Chinese medicine, takes a holistic view and advocates moderation, balance and harmony. Chinese herbal medicines aim to restore the five elements, wood, fire, earth, metal and water in balance, together with the forces of yin and yang. Yang expends energy; yin conserves it. Wood is the element specifically associated with the gallbladder.

The result of treatment with some Chinese herbal medicines in recent years has been damage to the kidneys, but this has often turned out to be due to the adulteration of the herb mixture with cheaper ingredients. Allergic reactions have also occurred. Chinese herbs are usually dried and this makes it more difficult to identify them. Chinese herbal teas are an acquired taste, but some people find a slow improvement in all types of symptom with TCM, while thousands in the West now take ginseng.

Western herbal medicines

The *Materia Medica*, compiled by Dioscorides, a Roman army doctor, contained some 600 remedies and Galen, also in the first century AD, added to them in his writings. Herbal folklore was the medicine of the common people in the Middle Ages, while Greek and Roman medical knowledge was confined to the monasteries. In the sixteenth century Paracelsus aimed at a scientific approach with *The Doctrine of Signatures*. Plants, by their appearance, were thought to indicate the diseases they might cure, such as Lungwort for chest problems.

In the eighteenth century scientific medicine started to take over and only in the American colonies were the old herbal remedies still used. The sparkling success of modern pharmaceutics is only now beginning to lose its gloss, and those afraid of side-effects or with 'green' leanings support modern herbalism. There are herbs, numbered in thousands, for every disease and every part of the body. Although you can just read the labels or get some guidance from a health store assistant, to get the best from herbal medicine – as with everything else – you need to consult an expert.

A herbal practitioner will select a mix to suit you, the individual's constitution and personality as well as the symptoms. Herbal treatments specifically recommended for gallstones include balmony, globe artichoke, rosemary, sage and dandelion. Infusions of marigold garlic drunk or taken in capsules, and tincture of devil's claw with celery seed are a tonic to the digestion, while slippery elm bark and marshmallow root calm it down after an upset. Aloe vera and meadowsweet either in capsules or as tea are generally soothing, as are most members of the umbellifera family: fennel, dill, cumin, caraway, anise and coriander. Cardamom, from the ginger family, clover and sage, chamomile and black horehound all suit some people with digestive troubles including gallstones.

Bilberry is believed to be good for stomachaches, also stone root and fringetree if you can find them. Heartburn is settled with angelica or lemon juice in apple cider. Spearmint and peppermint are generally useful in this area.

Homoeopathy

This complex, long-established, comprehensive system of medicine and treatment can be used for almost any disorder, but it is particularly efficacious for aches and pains associated with 'buried' psychological problems. It is also recommended for stomachache, indigestion, heartburn and colitis.

The homoeopathic principle of 'Like cures like' was known to the Greeks, but it was Samuel Hahnemann in the late eighteenth century who worked it out in detail and promoted it. He was reacting against the harsh medicines of the day, including leeches and purges. By experimenting on himself he reached this conclusion and founded the American Institute of Homoeopathy in 1848. *Nosodes* were remedies concocted by Hahnemann to counteract *miasms*, inherited weaknesses underlying all symptoms.

In the UK the fact that the Royal Family uses homoeopathic medicines enhances the medicines' acceptability despite the absence of a scientific basis for them. The current homoeopathic theory is that vital forces keep the body in health, until they are put under strain. Symptoms are regarded as evidence that the natural powers of self-healing are coming into play, and homoeopathic treatment, like much complementary medicine, seeks to rev up the body's defences rather than suppress unpleasant symptoms. The medicines tend to produce similar symptoms to those of the illness they are used to treat if appreciable doses are used.

Hahnemann discovered, he thought, that the more he diluted the medicines the more effective and the more specific they became. He called the dilution 'potentization'. At least it ensured that the treatment could cause no harm. As recently as 1988, Jacques Benveniste carried out experiments which seemed to show that even if not one molecule of the substance remained it could still affect living cells by having been there, leaving electromagnetic traces or footprints – a 'water memory'. No one has been able to replicate these findings.

Not many medical doctors go along with the theory, but a substantial number feel homoeopathy is worth a try if nothing else works.

Many homoeopathic practitioners are medically qualified but it is wise to have any unexplained symptoms checked out by your GP if you have a lay therapist.

Joanna

Joanna had the standard homoeopathic treatment. She was 35 and had endured a mixed bag of symptoms on and off for two or three years. She was convinced that her gallbladder was at fault but her GP thought it was biliary dyspepsia. Ultrasound had shown no stones, but she continued to have indigestion after a fatty meal, flatulence and headaches. At her insistence the doctor referred her to a homoeopathic colleague.

The first consultation lasted two hours – later sessions were shorter. Initially they went through Joanna's medical history and life history, her diet and lifestyle, her likes and dislikes. During the interview the practitioner was assessing her constitution, and put her down as a Lycopodium type – bright but psychologically insecure, and liable to problems in the digestive system. Each of the many types is known by the name of the appropriate remedy, in this case a plant. Joanna had to take it in the form of a tablet slipped under her tongue in a spoon – she was not supposed to handle it. The medicine was to be taken at least half-an-hour after a meal and she could not eat or drink anything for 15 minutes afterwards.

The taste was slightly sweet because the basic material of the tablet was lactose, milk sugar. During the course Joanna had to avoid anything with a strong smell or flavour – spicy foods, coffee, peppermint, menthol, tobacco, toothpaste and aromatherapy oils. At first she felt slightly worse, but this was a good sign, she was told. Some weeks, then a few months went by before Joanna was able to report a definite reduction in her symptoms. Her therapist said that this showed that the treatment had successfully stimulated her self-healing powers. No further treatment was needed unless or until new problems arose.

Great-grandmother's treatment

The Victorians knew all about what they called catarrh of the bile passages caused by stones, and more violent attacks with pain, vomiting and cold sweats – acute cholecystitis.

Treatment came under two heads: during the paroxysms of colic; and between attacks. In the first situation the urgent aim was to relieve the intense pain – using full doses of morphia. If morphia by mouth caused more vomiting, they gave it by injection. Another method was to put the patient in a warm bath and keep it topped up with hot water. Finally if this and the morphia did not work, the victim was anaesthetized with chloroform or ether. Surgery for acute appendicitis and cholecystitis came in at the turn of the century.

Between acute attacks the favourite medicine was Durande's mixture – three parts of ether to two of turpentine. It tasted so horrible that it had to be given in 'pearls' or capsules. The Germans swore by the Carlsbad waters for gallstones, while others recommended the great British standby, purgatives: castor oil, dandelion (taraxacum) and aqua regia. We should be thankful for the sophistication of modern surgery and modern drug therapy, but perhaps to have, as an extra, one of the gentler complementary therapies plus a chance to discuss how we feel is best of all.

13

Psychological aspects

Pain

Pain caused by gallstones is felt in the abdomen. Abdominal pain is a universal experience and one of the most primitive. Hardly has the baby emerged from his mother's womb, at the cost of some pain to her, than he is aware of sensations of varying degrees of unpleasantness in his own abdomen.

First comes plain hunger, then the painful stretching of stomach and gut from the air he has swallowed, followed by the blessed burp. Finally there is rising abdominal tension and the relief of passing a motion – all before he is a week old. None of us goes through life later without sometimes eating well but unwisely and earning the pain of indigestion, and we get muscle cramps from exercise. Women and girls expect some period pains. It is no surprise that a large proportion of patients in a GP's surgery come complaining of abdominal pain. It is outstripped only by back and head pain.

Emergencies such as acute appendicitis, acute cholecystitis or perforated ulcer are comparatively rare – most of them can only happen once in a person's lifetime. The diagnosis is usually straightforward, as is the treatment: in most cases it is surgical. What is much commoner and more likely to present a problem is persistent or recurrent moderate pain, with nothing dramatic to show for it. Tummy-aches are an everyday occurrence in children and in 90 per cent of those severe enough to be referred to a paediatric clinic the cause turns out to be emotional.

The surprising fact is that in both medical and surgical outpatient clinics for adults, among those sent by their doctors because of abdominal pain, only 15 patients in 100 are found to have any organic – that is, physical – disorder. In a major study only 48 patients in 2000 with abdominal pain had gallstone problems. Irritable bowel syndrome topped the list. A check five years later showed that only 2 per cent had developed a physical disorder in the interim.

Of the 85 per cent of patients with no evidence of physical disease the most frequent psychiatric diagnosis was depression – pain and depression are cousins – and the next commonest was chronic tension, an unremitting kind of anxiety that makes mild pain worse. Some of the men were heavy drinkers, which is halfway between a psychological and an organic problem. Pain, the key symptom, is a uniquely unpleasant psychological state, focused on one part of the body, in this case the abdomen. It is spiked with anxiety and an ominous sense of trouble to come. It is totally subjective. No one else can feel your pain, you cannot show it to anyone or even prove its existence. Virginia Woolf, when writing *On Being Ill*, remarked that 'language runs dry' when it comes to conveying what your personal pain is like. Churning, dragging, stabbing, gnawing, crushing and burning are all terms used to describe pain. Sometimes the choice of adjective tells more about the circumstances than the pain.

Tom

Tom was a big man, and it was not just muscle. He enjoyed good living and had not stinted himself – until now. He had only recently retired, early – at 55, and was surprised to find how lost he felt. He wondered if leisure really suited him. Then he found he did not fancy his usual 'full English' fried breakfast as he had previously. In fact his appetite dropped off altogether and a 'nagging' ache set in on the right side of his abdomen, sharpening into frank pain after a decent plateful of anything, however bland. He remembered an uncle who had suffered from gallstones (or was it gout?) and decided that he must have the same. He had no time for doctors and thought he could sort himself out.

Since eating was certain to give him pain, Tom cut it down to a minimum. What saved him, as he saw it, was that alcohol satisfied him and did not upset his stomach. His wife had been only too willing to cook anything he might fancy, but she only succeeded in irritating him. It was to escape her nagging that finally he went to see his GP and the detective work began. An ultrasound examination for gallstones, arranged at Tom's own suggestion, revealed two small stones in the gallbladder; they looked harmless. It was the liver enzyme tests were the give-away.

Tom's loss of appetite and the right-sided pain were due to alcoholic gastritis and early liver damage, respectively. The two little gallstones were irrelevant, although Tom liked to blame them for at least part of his problem. That he used the terms 'nagging' and 'wearing' to describe his abdominal discomfort reflected his resentment at his wife's frequent reminders of the dangers of drink. He did not appreciate his doctor's advice about cutting down, either.

What you need to be able to feel pain

You cannot feel pain if you are unconscious – the basis of anaesthesia for surgery or hypnosis in childbirth. It also requires your attention. In a car smash immediately after the impact, or playing in the Cup Final you do not notice any pain at the time: you need to turn your attention to what has happened to be able to feel it. The other side of the coin is your sharply focused mind when you are in the dentist's chair, or you see the needle about to prick your arm for a simple blood test. Pain is sharpened and magnified in these circumstances.

Finally, you must have learned the meaning of pain. Puppies brought up in isolation cages in which they experienced none of the minor pains of normal puppydom did not learn to avoid or shrink from harmful stimuli. They were curious about match flames and interested in pinpricks and did not associate them with harm or danger. They had not learned the primary meaning of pain and did not connect pain with tissue stress or damage as we do. Pavlov's dogs were taught that the pain of a mild electric shock would be followed by food. For them, the pain was worth the reward so they did not try to avoid it.

Both these animal experiments are applicable to human pain. We learn as children the response to pain that our parents demonstrate. A mother who makes a great fuss when her toddler falls over is teaching him to feel the pain to the maximum and fear it in the future – the reverse of the puppies' situation. Although the primary message of pain is of harm, it may have a compelling secondary meaning. For Pavlov's dogs this was food-on-the-way. For us, pain, itself a psychological state, can have many meanings. Those for abdominal pain in particular may be simple or subtle.

The secondary meanings of abdominal pain, which could be suspected of being due to gallstones, are all unconscious. They cover a wide and diverse range and include:

Comfort to come

A baby crying with colic receives the maximum attention, with comforting, affection, a feed or being carried around. This is surely recorded in his pre-verbal memory as a good experience. Similarly, in an older child or adult the drama and pain of an appendix operation may leave a memory of parents and friends being gratifyingly concerned and generous, linked with the pain. In either of these cases a wish for love and attention at a later date may be translated into abdominal pain – triggered by some disappointment or reverse.

Jill, Philip, Alice and Daphne all suffered from abdominal pains which puzzled their doctors. All four were suspected of having gallstones at one time or another, but in only one of them were stones responsible for the pain.

Guilt and expiation

Jill

Jill, aged 39, had three children. The third pregnancy was fraught, the result of a one-night error of judgement: her husband did not know that he was not the father. Jill had tried discreetly but unsuccessfully to bring on a miscarriage when she first realized she was pregnant. The child developed leukaemia when he was two, and Jill fell into a state of guilt and despair. She could not share her feelings openly with her husband, but presented an appearance of emotional calm – as though she did not care. Her abdominal pains started then, with sickness very like the morning sickness that had accompanied the pregnancy. Her doctor sent her for counselling, but she slipped into a depression and needed full psychiatric help. When the depression had been treated Jill's abdominal pain subsided. The little boy has responded to treatment.

We learn in childhood that being naughty means punishment means pain (not necessarily physical these days), and that wipes out the wrong-doing. It somehow felt right for Jill to have the abdominal pain and it took the edge off the depression.

Control over others, because of suffering

The highest religious example is that of Jesus Christ, but hunger-strikers like Bobby Sands had a great impact too. No one can feel comfortable in the face of someone else's suffering, particularly if they are in a position to do something about it.

Philip

Philip was 60 and had just retired, as was the company rule. June, his second wife, was 28 and they had been married for six years. She had been a junior staff nurse at the hospital when he was a patient with a perforated ulcer. At that time, he was a partner in a firm of merchant bankers whose name was a household word, and he had considerable influence. After this episode Philip had no more trouble from his ulcer, especially since the role of the helicobacter, the germ underlying many stomach problems, had been discovered.

Now, more than five years later, the abdominal pain came back, not as acutely as before, but much more frequently. Philip had not only lost his prestigious position, but at 60 he was no longer a star at tennis or squash and often had a stomach pain when June had arranged to play with friends of her own age. Of course, she did not go if he was not well, and Philip was truly distressed at being such a drag. He insisted on a full investigation of his pains, including a cholecystogram and ultrasound. His stomach, duodenum and biliary system were given the 'all clear' – to his mortification, and the episodes of pain continued.

The marriage did not prosper and it was through the sessions with Relate that it became obvious that Philip's pains were an unconscious ploy to keep June close at hand, and to recapture some of the loving care he had enjoyed when they first became acquainted. A rejigging of their lifestyle allowed freedom for June to do things with younger people, and for Philip to hone his skills at golf and bridge, while together they appreciated music, the theatre and travel. Philip's pains raise their heads now and again.

Retaining someone or something lost

When someone has died they may be kept alive in the bereaved person's mind by their developing the symptoms. Even when the loved one is alive you can feel the same pains or find yourself wanting to cough like the child or partner about whom you are worried. It brings you closer.

Alice

Alice's mother developed Alzheimer's disease prematurely and Alice was trapped. She was on an endless treadmill of bathing, dressing, clearing up and rescuing her from various predicaments

– like forgetting how to release the catch on the loo door. And throughout it all there were the old lady's constant complaints about her stomach-ache, her bowels and her bad nights. Alice dreaded coming home from work, wondering what disaster awaited. Yet her mother was very sweet at times and would say how lucky she was to have a daughter who would never put her in one of those horrid homes.

It was the double incontinence that did it. Worse, she took to hiding the results in the most unsuitable places – the linen cupboard, a vase and finally the fridge. Alice's GP arranged for the mother to move into a nursing home – but she promptly had a stroke and died. Alice was distraught. She had not had time to impress on the old lady that she still loved her just as much, and that it was only that she could not cope with the new difficulties ... The abdominal pains started almost immediately, quite sharp at times, but Alice found them curiously comforting. They made her feel closer to her mother, whether or not divided by death. Nevertheless, they seemed to be getting worse. Ordinary indigestion medicines, over-the-counter or on prescription, did not help.

At the hospital, where her GP referred her, a blood test showed a barely noticeable degree of jaundice, and ultrasound revealed a gallbladder full of stones. After the operation – cholecystectomy – Alice's pains never returned and she was able to mourn for her mother in the ordinary way.

Escape from responsibility or trouble

Escape via pain, which is conveniently invisible, can be very attractive. 'Monday morning tummy-ache' is a well-established method of escaping school. If it works, however innocently, it prepares the ground for incapacitating abdominal pains when there are problems at work.

Daphne

Daphne had been one of those children who often had a tummy-ache. They had labelled it 'abdominal migraine' at one time, but it always cropped up on a school day, and usually when there was French on the timetable. Her mother was called to the school to take her home although she did not have a temperature and she was not sick, because she looked so poorly. She was usually well enough to see her favourite television programme in the afternoon. When Daphne's periods started, she was one of the unfortunates who get dysmenorrhoea, but now she was old enough for the school to send her home in a taxi.

After school and college Daphne, who had grown very pretty, had a PA job with a recording firm. Her boss, a man of 50, was understanding when Daphne had a bout of abdominal pain (it was not her periods now), and she was easily able to arrange time off to go to the doctor and incidentally fit in a little shopping. The doctor liked her too, and would give her a certificate if she needed a longer time in which to get better. The only person who did not sympathize was the girl who had to take on Daphne's work as well as her own when Daphne was ill. There was no question of Daphne 'putting on' her symptoms. She felt the pain and nausea, and she looked very pale. The reason for the symptoms may not have been physical, but how she felt was genuine. The pallor was part of it.

The skin reflects both organic illness and emotional states. You may blush with embarrassment, go purple with rage or ashy white with shock, anxiety or unhappiness. Daphne will probably always have a propensity to get a pain when some stress or difficulty crops up, but an assertiveness course helped a little. Sometimes pain can be convenient in legitimizing selfishness, rudeness or not pulling one's weight – an excuse for unacceptable behaviour that no one can argue with.

Communicating distress or need

Pain and distress go hand in hand. It is an automatic reaction for us to cry out if we are in pain before we have learned to express ourselves verbally. If a small child is tearful we are likely to ask: 'Where does it hurt?' As adults we can suffer emotional pain and have emotional needs, but most of us find it much easier to say we have got a pain or some other physical symptom, preferably with a bruise or a cut to show for it, than to admit, for example, that we are in distress over rejection by a lover. What we are seeking in such circumstances is to be comforted and reassured that someone cares about us. Pain brings this response from other people, even those we barely know.

Alexithymia: it may be the Englishman's disease, but women can have it too. It is an inability, perhaps because of a rigid upbringing, to express emotion. This may be related to the difficulty most of us have in finding words to describe our particular pain. It is a block on talking about our feelings, however harrowing, heart-breaking or fearful. Good feelings, like those of love, may also be side-tracked into euphemisms by an alexithyme.

Rodney

Rodney was 33. His father had been in the Army and he had been brought up in a series of army camps, with frequent changes of school. He was never sure what his values should be, except for the general one about a stiff upper lip. At 29 he married a beautiful girl and loved her with all his heart. It was when she was expecting twins and there were problems with her blood pressure, that Rodney's abdominal pains began. There had been both liver and gallbladder disorders among his relatives, largely because, like many Army men, they drank enthusiastically.

Rodney's proposal of marriage had run something like this – 'What about it, old girl?' Fortunately Esme had understood him. In the current situation he gave no indication that he was in a blind panic lest something should go seriously wrong – and she would die. Apart from bitter complaints about his pain he maintained a bluff, gruff manner and seemed heartlessly unconcerned about his wife. The Army surgeons, men of action, could find nothing they could excise from Rodney or subdue with drugs. There was no sign of a liver disorder or gallstones.

Rodney's pain gradually improved after the babies were born and their mother was blooming, if tired. No abdominal disease developed. The trickcyclist, as Rodney called him, suggested that this had been a case of the Couvade syndrome: pains, usually in the abdomen, affecting men whose wives are going through worrying pregnancies. If Rodney had not been alexithymic he could have discussed his fears with the obstetrician looking after Esme, and his distress and the pain it produced would have been defused to large extent by explanation.

Some people are accident-prone – you must have met one or two – while others are pain-prone. Instead of the odd twinge after an injury, or a touch of indigestion, which another person would ignore, the pain-prone one concentrates on it, broods over it, worries about it and it gets worse. The abdomen is one of the commonest sites.

The one thing pain-prone people have in common is that their early relationships were bound up with pain and suffering. It may have been a parent, a grandparent or someone else close whose life was so full of pain that the whole family lived through it and round it. This becomes the scene in which the pain-prone person feels most at home, later.

Mandy

When Mandy was growing up and finding her own identity, her grandmother, a woman of 70, came to live with Mandy's parents. Unhappily she developed a cancer of the rectum and went through major surgery leaving her with a colostomy. She kept going for several years, but then she was found to have secondaries in her liver. At this stage she had a great deal of pain, and died quite soon afterwards.

Mandy became liable to abdominal pains whenever she was put under extra strain, from her GCSEs onwards, and often when she was away from home. If someone in Mandy's situation is alexithymic, emotions can build up and finally overflow with a flood of pent-up pain from a minor trigger. Mandy's doctor had felt sure that some medical disaster – perhaps an ectopic pregnancy – had taken place, but there was never anything physically wrong to account for her pain.

Where you feel the pain

Because of the spaced-out nerve supply, and the way the nerves are shared, pain in the abdomen is a poor guide to the situation inside. Nevertheless its location can be significant. Mild to moderate central or generalized pain is common and may be due to either a physical or a psychological cause. Psychological pain is especially likely to be felt where there has been pain previously, for instance in the appendix area when the appendix has long gone, or in the pelvic area after some gynaecological problem.

For women more than men psychologically mediated pains in the abdomen are often a reaction to concern about sexual matters. Period pains, which may be purely physical but often have an emotional aspect, may have a beneficial side-effect. They can strengthen the bonds of friendship between young teenage girls, and provide some fellow feeling, as females together, between mothers and daughters. Pain can also be experienced 'in just the same place' as someone important in your life. Conflict or separation tend to bring this on.

Psychiatric disorders

Any of the ordinary psychiatric disorders can become associated with abdominal pain. They include:

- depression: neurotic, the usual type, or very severe – psychotic;
- chronic tension;
- anxiety states, ranging from worry to stark panic;
- conversion hysteria and hypochondriasis;
- schizophrenia.

The important trick is to recognize a psychological disorder when it is at the root of the physical symptoms. One curious fact, which is logical if you think it through, is that pain which is caused by an emotional disturbance does not respond to chemical treatment. It is not doused out by full doses of powerful painkillers – you become drowsy before the pain eases.

Depression

This is a term that we bandy about casually yet it can cause the most intense suffering. It is almost the only illness which makes the victim so wretched that he or she contemplates suicide. Pain can be a life-saver since it provides some protection from the full force of emotional misery. It is a sanity-saving reflex in clinical depression that enhances a trivial pain into something too severe to be ignored, diverting some of the negative thoughts into different channels. It is important for your doctor, if not you, to spot the clues that tell when you have a depressive illness.

Abdominal pain, which may be blamed on 'silent' gallstones, is particularly likely in depression due to a loss or disappointment. The terms 'womb-dropping' and 'that sinking feeling' refer to this.

Gillian

Gillian was 45 when the wearying, non-stop aching started plaguing her. The trigger had been the double whammy of her father's death in Australia and being turned down for a headship, when she thought she stood a good chance. She did not tell the doctor all this, nor about the depression she had when she was a student – after all, it was a quarter of a century ago. What she did tell him was about the pain, continuing relentlessly regardless of meals, and that she had lost her appetite.

The excellent stomach drugs available nowadays did not touch Gillian's constant ache, any more than the standard analgesics. She was losing weight, unsurprising with her lack of interest in food, and waking in the small hours feeling dreadful. All her vitality seemed to have been siphoned off; she could not concentrate at work, nor feel interested in the family, sex or friends. It was at this point that the GP decided to try her on amitriptyline, an old-fashioned antidepressant which has made a recent comeback as a treatment for intractable pain.

After a few weeks of a dry mouth and disappointment at her lack of improvement, Gillian's pain and her mood lightened fractionally. The doctor then recognized that she was depressed, changed her medication to one of the newer SSRI (Selective Serotonin Re-uptake Inhibitor) antidepressants and referred her to the practice counsellor. Gillian was able to talk through her two losses and recovered completely within four or five months.

The depressive clues were her early history of depression; her loss of appetite and weight; poor sleep; loss of interest, concentration and libido; and a generally negative mood.

Chronic tension

This is a very common psychological state in these peaceless, stress-filled times. It causes muscle aches and painful spasms in the back and shoulders – and also in the gut. This last produces pain, stomach gurgles – and any or all of the symptoms of irritable colon (see p. 40) or of dyspepsia – or of both. Tension and anxiety make you acutely aware of abdominal discomfort, which becomes unendurably exhausting, while moderate pain is elevated to severe. Talking with a therapist is the safest treatment, but the Valium-type drugs are useful for a quick – temporary – fix. The danger is that used even for a week or two, they become addictive. The same applies to alcohol, a special trap for those who are chronically tense.

Hysterical conversion

This is nothing to do with being neurotically excitable, but is very like the situation in depression. Physical pain, in this case in the abdomen, and which could have been suspected of being due to gallstones, occurs in place of obvious psychological distress. This is usually bound up with conflict in a relationship and you may not want everyone to know what you are feeling. Doctors may find it puzzling that you seem calm but complain of pain for which they cannot find a physical explanation. It is essential, when you have unexplained pain, to review all the worries, stresses and upsetting events you have had in the last six months.

One of the most dismal situations is when you have pain or other symptoms and the doctor says 'There's nothing wrong.' This is a lie and an insult. It is so obviously untrue that you may feel that you are being fobbed off because he suspects a cancer and does not want to tell you. This is extremely unlikely these days, but such worrying thoughts can haunt you. They need dealing with sympathetically and more thoroughly than is possible in the standard three-minute GP consultation. If there is any question of your having a psychological factor in your symptoms you need a counsellor, a clinical psychologist, a psychotherapist or a psychiatrist to help you sort it out. The type of helper depends on which you find most acceptable.

What you can do to help yourself

Do not go on taking medicines out of politeness to your doctor if you find they are not helping you. Explain the situation. The drugs themselves are likely to upset your digestive and biliary systems if you continue on them indefinitely.

Try to live as normal a life as possible while you are waiting for your symptoms to subside. This difficult process pays off in that, as you do recover, you are already partway there. Do not stop work for longer than you must, so that you have not too many threads to pick up.

Especially, go out of your way to keep in contact with your friends, even if you cannot contribute much, and do talk about anything and everything except your physical symptoms.

Finally: do not feel disheartened. Emotional upsets and disorders are not permanent.

Useful addresses

UK

British Liver Trust

Ransomes Europark
Ipswich IP3 9QG
Tel: 01473 276326
Fax: 01473 276327
Information line: 0808 800 1000
http://www.britishlivertrust.org.uk

Children's Liver Disease Foundation

40–42 Stoke Road
Guildford GU1 4HS
Tel: 01483 300565
Fax: 01483 300530

USA

American Liver Foundation

75 Maiden Lane
Suite 603
New York
NY 10038
1–800–GO LIVER (465–4837)
http://gi.ucsf.edu/alf.html

Canada

Canadian Liver Foundation

Suite 310, 1320 Yonge Street
Toronto
Ontario M4T 1X2
Tel: (416) 964 1953
Fax: (416) 964 0024

Germany

Deutsche Leberhelfe e.V.

Gesmolden Strasse 27
D–4520
Mellel
Germany
Tel: (05422) 6568
Fax: (05422) 44499

Index